RADICAL RADIANCE

RADICAL
RADIANCE

12 Weeks of Self-Love Rituals
to Manifest Abundance,
Beauty, and Joy

ANGELA JIA KIM

ST. MARTIN'S
ESSENTIALS
NEW YORK

First published in the United States by St. Martin's Essentials, an imprint of St. Martin's Publishing Group

www.stmartins.com

Design by Susan Walsh
Graphics courtesy of Savor Beauty, designed by Escarla Abreu.

The Library of Congress Cataloging-in-Publication Data is available upon request.

ISBN 978-1-250-85319-6 (paper over board)
ISBN 978-1-250-81215-5 (ebook)

Our books may be purchased in bulk for promotional, educational, or business use. Please contact your local bookseller or the Macmillan Corporate and Premium Sales Department at 1-800-221-7945, extension 5442, or by email at MacmillanSpecialMarkets@macmillan.com.

First Edition: 2022

10   9   8   7   6   5   4   3   2   1

Dedicated to you, radiant soul

CONTENTS

INTRODUCTION
The Self-Love Radiance

We all know what it's like to feel stressed, drained, overwhelmed, and downright dull—in other words, the opposite of radiant. In fact, while I was writing this book, our entire world was experiencing a life-changing pandemic that forced us to spend countless hours alone. Like it or not, this gave us a plethora of time to examine ourselves, on the inside and out.

So tell me: do you like what you see and love who you are?

I'm Angela Jia Kim—a retired concert pianist, beauty entrepreneur, single mom, and New Yorker. I've written the book you're holding in your hands because I've come to believe that the blending of inner and outer radiance—a new and improved version of self-care—is the greatest act of self-love that you can practice. Self-love starts with knowing *who you are* so that you can radiate your authentic beauty, brilliance, and balance. Perhaps you're successful at work, have a loving family, or think your partner is ideal; but without self-love, factors like burnout, stress, and the daily blues can sabotage your best intentions.

Enter: Radical Radiance.

Why do I call this Radical Radiance? People always think "radical" means "extreme," but the word actually comes from the Latin word *radix,* meaning "root." We are going to go to the root of who you are and do deep inner work on your soul's essence for a visible vibrant glow. My own discovery of radiant self-love began with skincare, but it goes further and deeper than that. My Korean mother taught me to treat my skin like the most expensive silk on earth, which is a beautiful first step toward teaching self-love. The skin needs exfoliation, detoxification, purification, and nourishment—as do the deepest and most sacred parts of your soul. The good news is, my experience and research with thousands of women have shown me that everyone has the ability to discover inner and outer radiance. When you illuminate your most authentic self that shines from every pore of your being, you create a magnetic force that's irresistible and attractive. Together, we'll nourish your glow to bring about all the abundance, love, and joy that you not only crave, but deserve.

I have been studying radiance my entire adult life as a performer and now as the founder of a skincare and spa brand. I teach thousands of women the Korean philosophy of always going to the *root* cause of their skin issues instead of heaping on makeup to cover what they perceive as flaws. It's the same process with your soul, but because it's invisible to you, it's easy to ignore root issues and cover blockages with self-sabotage. We *think* our inner energy is invisible to others even though it's in and around us, but it affects the way we live, how we manifest, and how we connect with ourselves and others.

To get to the root, then, we need to prioritize self-love and cultivate rituals to nourish our inner radiance. In this book, we will carve out time for self-love adventures, self-care sabbaticals, exploration playdates, inspiration getaways, creativity excursions, and frequency equilibriums. We will also use everyday emotions to remind us to nourish our inner radiance with self-love. When we feel down, irritated, upset, angry, stressed, or anxious, this serves as a reminder that our soul craves love as much as the body needs water. Self-love is not selfish, nor is it vain. It's the most generous act of care that we can do for ourselves, our lovers, families, and friends. In the warmth of self-love, our authentic being lights up and kindles love for others. This ultimately allows us to give from a cup that overflows with a lit-from-within quality.

A Bit About Me

So how did my personal philosophies and teachings come to be? At my foundation, I absorbed the traits I admire most in my parents. My dad, who passed away when I was thirteen years old, epitomized productivity and came from a long line of ancestors who manifested tremendous success in Korea and the United States. My mom had four sisters, all of whom embodied "skincare is self-care," a Korean beauty manifesto. Together, I managed to marry Dad's drive and Mom's beauty philosophies to create a multimillion-dollar business called Savor Beauty + Spa, based in Manhattan.

Though I was groomed to become a concert pianist from the age of three, it took many more years to stumble on my true calling as an entrepreneur and women's thought leader. One of my "Aha!" moments happened while on tour before a piano performance; I put a "natural" lotion on my body and broke out into horrible hives in front of hundreds of people. It was a humiliating experience. After the recital, I saw that the ingredients were full of chemicals. As a fun hobby and antidote to my problem, I decided to start making creams and beauty oils in my kitchen. As I've mentioned, if my dad's family taught me work ethic, my mom taught me to love skincare. She was always using beautiful face creams sent to her from Seoul that were made from pigeon poop, silkworm cocoons, and gold flecks. I knew, however, that there were a lot of toxic ingredients in these formulas. Because I was concerned about possible carcinogens and overall health, I wanted her to use antiaging skincare that was effective *and* organic.

Making creams in my kitchen turned out to not only be

healing for my skin, but also for my soul. For the first time in my life, I was allowed to make mistakes without serious consequences. All of my life at the piano, I had my teachers around me, correcting my errors and coaching me to play with perfection. During my solo piano career, I spent countless hours practicing passages over and over to be "perfect" on stage. If I did not perform optimally, I felt that too much was on the line: audience disappointment, criticism from all directions, and a dip in my self-worth.

Creating skincare, however, felt freeing. I could mess up, clean up, and start over. Being a concert pianist taught me dedication, perseverance, grit, and to strive for excellence—traits I applied to my skincare process but without the added pressure. After about a thousand tries (seriously), and with my mom as my muse, I began giving my creations as gifts to friends, who then bought them as gifts for their friends. My mom also gave them to her sisters, who loved the creams. As it turns out, I'd concocted the perfect face cream that even a Korean woman would covet!

As I became an "accidental entrepreneur," I simultaneously burned out from the pursuit of perfection as a pianist. While pregnant with my daughter, Sienna, I gave my last performance, closed the piano lid, and realized that I craved rejuvenation. One month after I gave birth, I felt a sudden surge of creative energy. I opened a little holiday pop-up shop to showcase my skincare in Bryant Park, and while breastfeeding, I learned my very first business lesson: how to sell. At first, it felt humiliating. I was used to being courted as the star of the show, and now I was the cosmetics girl who was being rejected over and over again. There were many days that I'd retreat into my little kiosk and cry while hugging my little one-month-old daughter. I was lucky to have the support of Marc, my then husband, who encouraged me to keep going even when I felt like quitting. Ultimately, with a lot of perseverance, support, and determination, I eventually sold around $40,000 in creams that season, which gave me the confidence to open my first retail store and, eventually, a boutique spa in the West Village.

Going from pianist to entrepreneur proved challenging. With not enough money to open my first store (I put $60,000 on my credit cards), zero connections, and barely any experience, I felt just as lonely as I did as a solo musician. Only this time, I had mounting bills and new stresses. I didn't have the proper funds or the time to go to business school, so I decided to gather other women in the same boat so that we could learn from each other. I put a post on Craigslist for a gathering in my living room, and women from all over New York City came and exchanged ideas, thoughts, and support. The group kept growing, and eventually it became a business organization called Savor the Success, which had hundreds of members, support circles, and virtual content to help women grow their businesses. These were women who wanted to launch their own businesses, and they wanted to learn from me, as they saw my beauty business grow from a hobby to a small company.

The skills I learned as a pianist—going from the practice room to the performance hall—took vision, discipline, courage, and resilience. These were the transferable skills that helped me launch my skincare business. I possessed a positive, upbeat, and inspired creative energy that other women were attracted to, and they wanted to learn the manifestation process from me. This is how I began hosting hundreds of manifesting workshops and conferences, and created a popular planner (now called *Savor Beauty Planner: My Next 90 Days*) that reflected many of the manifesting philosophies taught to me by my dad. This planner has helped over one hundred thousand women use their creative force to dream up and accomplish goals. The organizer was and continues to be the first of its kind to also help women focus on planning self-care every day.

I reached a point where I was spreading myself so thin, however, that I soon realized that I'd lost myself again, and I did not know how to handle the pressure of running two companies with employees and members—plus being an attentive mom to my young daughter, who needed me. My work ethic had turned into "workaholism." I fell into a people-pleasing trap, and the familiar signs of burnout dimmed my light once again. It looked from the outside as though I was on top of the world. It seemed so glamorous and successful, but something felt *very* wrong. It was again clear that I needed to make a significant lifestyle change. So in 2018, with a thriving business and substantial platform under my belt, I made the heart-wrenching decision to let go of Savor the Success, the women's entrepreneur organization, and focus solely on Savor Beauty and my employees. I knew that I needed to give back from a place of more authenticity and less approval. Like most scary decisions, I didn't know what would happen, but I took small steps, listened to my intuition, and the right answers revealed themselves. I then began to focus more on myself and my own needs, through daily self-exploration and self-love rituals. I found that feeding myself and my soul in these ways gave me the balance and nourishment that I'd been craving all along.

The self-love rituals that you'll find in the following pages are a collection of a lifetime of research, formulation, and trial-and-error experimentation. They are a culmination of everything I learned as a musician, entrepreneur, mom, lover, and mentor to teach countless women how to authentically access and celebrate their inner and outer beauty.

In 2020, I faced a triple whammy of challenges: the pandemic, a divorce, and the mandated shutdown of my spas for nearly six months. It was devastating to be stripped of the things that, years ago, I thought made me matter, the images that I thought made me worthy, and the happy wife / successful entrepreneur labels that I thought made me shine. What I discovered through the beauty of self-love (the new and improved version of self-care), however, is that I was okay *without* all these labels and masks. The miracles that came from consistently nourishing my radiance helped our e-commerce business to flourish and the divorce to end amicably (my ex is one of my good friends, to this day). And even though I found the shutdown one of the most lonely times in our history—as it was for many—I continued to feel whole and radiant.

When the pandemic began, New York City became a ghost town, and as a newly single mom, I stayed home like everyone else. I decided to create the twelve-week self-love program in this book. I even added to the soul-care rituals I'd planned to include, since I was now using and tweaking them to help me navigate my new reality with gratitude and grace. I hope the end result helps you through a re-vealing, transformative, and fun process that allows you to radiate an inner and outer beauty that is authentically you and yours.

How to Use This Book

Radical Radiance is dedicated to three months of self-love ritu-als and divided into twelve themed weeks. In my experience, after having led hundreds of women through my ninety-day Savor Success Circles programs using *Savor Beauty Planner: My Next 90 Days,* I've learned that we can focus on *anything* for ninety days. This is long enough to make a difference and short enough for you to change course, if needed.

As you work through the chapters, I recommend that you go in consecutive order since one week builds on the next. Each week also includes a few rituals for you to practice when you feel inspired; feel free to infuse one or two (or all) of them into your day and build from there. You can also customize the rituals to support your unique needs. Practice makes progress!

As you read through the book, you may also get the impression that I have everything pulled together, wrapped with a pretty, polished bow. One of my friends even called me the other day and said, "What am I doing wrong? Did I pull the short straw, or am I praying to the wrong gods? You seem to have it all figured out. What are your secrets?" Trust me, I have my fair share of down days, whether it's navigating business challenges (the spa rebuild post-COVID has been as daunting as the mandated shutdown) or family growing pains. The answer to my friend was that in times of trouble, I always return to the bite-size and doable rituals in this book. You can do one of them, do all of them, come back to them, repeat them, curate them, customize them.

PRO TIP: I like to do most of my rituals at a beauty altar to feel uplifted and inspired. Rebecca Casciano, founder of The Sacred Beauty Collective, teaches how to create a designated space to practice inner and outer beauty rituals. Rebecca says, "To set up a beauty altar, you need a mirror, tabletop area, and decent lighting. Then add sacred objects, such as crystals, shells, and favorite photos of yourself, a family member, and/or your beauty muse. I like to have plants, flowers, candles, and incense on the altar or nearby, which I light before my makeup application. I believe that applying our makeup with intention can elevate it from a mundane beauty routine to a gorgeous self-love ritual!" I couldn't agree more, and I also like to say empowering affirmations, listen to an inspiring talk, or just meditate and *be*.

Finally, I'd like you to prioritize self-love by *planning* to do the rituals rather than haphazardly squeezing them into your hectic day. Bake the rituals into your schedule by creating GCal reminders or using a planner of choice. Make yourself a priority. If you'd like to use the *Savor Beauty Planner: My Next 90 Days* as a complementary organizer to this program, you can find it at savorbeautyplanner.com. You will also notice that many of the rituals ask you to use optional beauty products, accessories, crystals, sticky notes, and pens. The ones you choose are entirely up to you and your preferences. You can find a lot of these products online and some of them at savorbeauty.com.

Ready to get started? Let's roll up our sleeves and get to work, beauty!

Week 1

START WITH YOUR SKIN

There's an old saying that goes, "As above so below, and so below as above." Throughout time, astrologers have used this adage to explain that the stars and earth are inextricably linked in more ways than we could ever imagine: everything is interconnected. And in ancient Korean times specifically, the body and spirit were also considered one; it was believed that inner happiness was reflected on our faces and bodies. This may explain why Korean women have been working on their skin's radiance from as far back as AD 918, when natural concoctions from safflower, apricot, and peach oils were used to remove age spots and add a glossy sheen to the skin.

My Korean mom was my muse when I began making lotions and potions in my kitchen as a hobby, before it turned into a bona fide skincare business. At seventy-something years old, Mom is proof that following a skincare regimen for long-lasting results is a marathon, not a sprint. After I created Savor Beauty's signature Truffle Face Cream, she said, "Angie-ah, now my skin needs a *syrup* to put under the cream. Can you make one?" She meant "serum," of course, and she would massage the potion I made onto her face, neck, and décolletage. Without knowing it, Mom was teaching me how to layer love onto my skin. Whenever she walks into the Savor Beauty spas in New York City, the entire team stops to get a glimpse of her radiance. The aestheticians study her face under the magnifying lamp and admire her skin's youthful elasticity, refined pores, and smooth luminosity.

"Treat your skin like the most expensive silk," my mom would always preach. As a child, I'd marvel at her vanity table, filled with new creams that her sisters had sent to her from Korea: one with gold flecks, another with silkworm cocoons, and yet another with exotic seaweed. All of them promised to make her skin smooth like silk, creamy like milk, and clear like water.

Fast-forward twenty years: my mom is now a grandma who has taken Sienna, my daughter, under her skin-radiance wing. Recently, as my mom was serving my daughter and nephew fruit snacks she had prepared, she said, "Sienna, your skin is too dry. You have to eat more fruit. See, look at Zachie." She pointed to my two-year-old nephew. "His face is shiny because he eats a lot of fruit," said my mom, smiling brightly at him, her new skincare prodigy.

Shiny. Radiant. And to think, I spent my teenage years rebelling against Mom's direction and instead covering up a big part of my Korean culture with alcohol toners, rough facial scrubs, and powder. While Western wisdom uses all kinds of skincare to mattify the skin and heavy makeup to hide blemishes, my mom's and aunts' Eastern philosophy involved timeless beauty rituals to achieve luminosity and glow. Radiating a translucent complexion is not something we can earn overnight—it requires layering love and care, every day, onto the skin to reveal a naturally radiant and refined texture. Just as we care for our inner essence, we also need to care for our outer selves. I believe their essences are intertwined, as you'll learn in this book.

Skincare is where I began my discovery of radiant self-love, but it goes further and deeper than that, as you will see. It is the symbolic first lesson in *Radical Radiance* to treat the skin like the most expensive silk on earth, as Mom would say—an honor we'll later apply to the soul.

Cleanse Your Face Every Night

Beauty is the radiance of your soul.
—Asad Meah, CEO and founder, Awaken the Greatness Within

Have you ever heard of The FlyLady? That's the nickname given to Marla Cilley, a home-organization coach who teaches her clients how to eliminate clutter with baby-step routines. I discovered her in my twenties, and while I learned a lot from this expert, she had one piece of advice that changed my life forever: shine your sink before going to bed every night. The concept is to go to bed feeling accomplished and wake up feeling good to be greeted by a shiny sink. This small habit sets the foundation for many other little habits that string together simple routines to help the day run smoothly. Ever since I committed to going to bed with a shining sink over twenty years ago, it set the foundation for a string of rituals that helped me to go from living in complete mayhem to maintaining a minimalist, sparkling home.

When I wanted to shine from the inside out, I took a page from The FlyLady's philosophy on baby steps and did something small and simple that changed everything for me in a different way: I began a nightly facial double-cleansing ritual. I continued to shine my sink, but now I was intent on shining my face, too. Don't get me wrong—I always washed my face, and it's something my mom ingrained in me since I was young. "Did you *sesu* (wash your face), Angie-ah?" she would ask from the other room. To appease her, I spent many years scrubbing my face with an apricot scrub and splashing water everywhere to take it off as fast as possible.

It wasn't until I viewed washing my face as an enjoyable ritual, rather than as a one-more-thing-I-must-do chore, that I began to understand the profoundness of this small act of supreme self-care. I breathed in the cleanser's aroma, massaged away the day's tension, softened the skin, and swept away dirt and toxins. Slowing down each evening felt surprisingly good, and over time, I craved more feel-good rituals. This was the beginning of my self-love journey.

We will create a fresh foundation for you, too, as we walk a new and radically radiant path together. Ending every night with a face-cleansing ritual will renew and replenish your skin and soul. This is the first daily ritual that you will infuse into your life as a symbol of self-love through sunshine and storms, good days and bad. And the best part? It only takes *one minute.* One minute to remind yourself, *"I matter."* Nightly cleansings will lay the foundation for many other little rituals that we'll string together for a lifestyle of Radical Radiance.

Beginning our self-love program with a nightly face-cleansing ritual is restorative because you're paying attention to yourself at the most basic, physical level. It grounds you in your skin and body with a calming, rhythmic energy as you wash away the day's grime. It also primes the brain (and complexion) for bedtime, so you wake up feeling good. And when you feel good, you look good.

Here's what can happen when you go to bed without washing your face:

- Free radicals sit overnight on your skin and break down your collagen and elastin, leading to fine lines and wrinkles.
- Sebum (oily substance) and sweat build up overnight, which leads to clogged pores and breakouts.

- The day's makeup, pollution, and bacteria settle into pores, making them appear larger.
- You don't feel your best in the morning when you wake up to a dry and dull complexion.

Good skin starts with clean skin, but not the "squeaky clean" kind. Too many people believe their face needs to feel dry after cleansing, but that's just stripping the skin of its nourishing barrier. We need to rewire our brains around what clean skin truly is: dewy and nourished, not stiff and tight, a metaphor we will later apply to soul-care. I love using a double-cleansing technique, a thorough Korean ritual, to achieve radiant, clear skin. The alluring aromas, sense of touch, and sound of water help me go to bed feeling nourished and replenished.

RITUAL: Nightly Double-Cleanse

To set your self-love foundation, using this nourishing evening* cleanse

---

*You can wash your face in the morning, too! I personally do an oil cleanse in the shower every morning because I have dry skin. For oily skin types, a thorough cleansing ritual may be necessary. Make sure to listen to your skin needs and cleanse accordingly. If in doubt, consult an aesthetician or dermatologist.

Time: 1–3 minutes

Ingredients: Cleansing oil and water-based cleanser (or cleanser of choice), clean towel

Optional Upgrades: Essential oil of choice

Notes: If you have oily skin, contrary to what you might think (or have been told for years), oil cleansers have the power to dissolve oil, unlike any other cleanser ingredient. It's true! Oil attracts oil and can dissolve sebum and dirt without stripping the skin of its natural oils.

1. **Prime.** Create a beautiful spa-like environment in your bathroom for this nightly cleansing ritual. I like to organize my beauty products on my sink in a minimalist fashion.

2. **Sanitize.** Wash your hands with soap to avoid putting dirt or bacteria onto your face. I run warm water and put 1–3 drops of an essential oil in the sink for a calming effect.

3. **Observe.** Look into the mirror and examine the baby hairs on your face. Which way do they naturally grow? You'll want to apply cleansing products with your fingertips using gentle, circular motions going in the opposite direction of your hair growth. This allows you to get into every nook and cranny for a thorough cleanse.

4. **Cleanse.** Warm several drops of a cleansing oil

between your clean fingers. Apply it to your face with your fingertips in circular motions to melt off the day's makeup. Oil cleansing will help pull out the dirt and grime that accumulates in your pores to avoid bacterial growth, blemishes, and irritation. If you have drier skin and are using an all-natural oil cleanser, consider leaving it on a little longer to hydrate and nourish the skin.

5. Layer. Layer a water-based cleanser on top of the oil cleanser, also in circular motions. This helps sweep away the day's dirt and grime, too. Enjoy the aroma and the way your skin feels under your fingertips.

6. Cleanse. Gently wash off the cleansers with warm water. I like to keep a drawer full of freshly laundered face towels nearby so that I can use a new one each day to pat the skin dry.

7. Appreciate. Use this time to affirm what makes you feel radiant. If you find it challenging to compliment yourself, it can be easier to use *"I'm grateful for . . ."* statements to show appreciation for your natural beauty.

"I am grateful for my cleansed skin."
"I feel grounded and clear."
"My skin feels smooth and hydrated."
"I love feeling radiant and glowing."

Savor this simple act of supreme self-care; it's the foundation for radical skin and soul radiance.

Tone to Brighten and Hydrate

True beauty in an [individual] is reflected in [their] soul.
—Audrey Hepburn, actress

I was always so intrigued by my mom's toners and essences. In Korea, an essence is like the love child of a toner and serum—a lightweight layer of hydration. My mom would take a fluffy white cotton ball and moisten it with a rose-colored essence and then softly sweep it upward on her skin. My favorite part was watching her repeat the upward strokes on her neck, décolletage, and back up onto her face until her skin glistened and beamed with moisture. I wanted to copy her, but during my teen years, I coveted the Americanized matte look. So I used an astringent toner and marveled at how breezy and dry my skin felt afterward. My mom always scolded me: "Angie-ah, your face looks drier now! This is not how to care for your skin. Your face should shine."

In college, I dropped the toner from my end-of-day routine. After practicing piano for eight hours, studying for exams, and socializing with friends, it felt like an unnecessary, time-consuming step. True enough, one of the most commonly asked questions that we get at Savor Beauty + Spa is, "Why do I need to tone; what is its purpose?" Toners have recently experienced a stunning renaissance, transforming from an unnecessary drying step to skincare's essential hydration station. In the past, toners contained drying alcohol or witch hazel, which strip the skin of youthful oils. The newer generation of toners contains nourishing, rebalancing, and hydrating ingredients to benefit oily *and* dry skin. Once I understood the inner workings of what a nonalcohol toner does for the skin, it became a staple in my beauty rituals.

After a thorough double cleanse, a toner balances the skin's pH for a juicy, hydrated, and healthy complexion. When you wash your face, the skin's pH balance can become out of whack, but toners help bring it back to a balanced 5.5 pH to work at its optimal level. If the skin is thrown off-balance, this can lead to sensitivity, wrinkles, inflammation, or breakouts.

My favorite types of toners are naturally derived hydrosols that wake up your complexion, quench parched pores, and provide skin-loving nutrients. A hydrosol combines the concept of a toner and essence into one. Hydrosols are tonics that are produced when flowers and plants are distilled. This "flower water" serves the toner's purpose to prep the skin for moisturizers and the essence's purpose to lightly hydrate. It's alcohol-free, replenishing, and packed with nutrients, antioxidants, and vitamins. You can find different flower and plant hydrosols, depending on your skin concern.

As I created Savor Beauty's toners, I didn't want customers to have to take the extra step of dipping a cotton ball into an essence, because I wanted them to be able to freshen up in a New York minute. Personally, I craved a face mist to carry around in my bag to revive me throughout the day—before a presentation, after yoga, or during a phone meeting. I experimented by putting hydrosols into a mister, and voilà—I had my multitasking and portable beauty BFF.

In the morning, I often wake up with parched pores. The following Daily Morning Mist ritual is my go-to solution (along with Turkish coffee and a fig) to both wake up my body and open my skin pores to drink up the hydration goodness.

RITUAL: Daily Morning Mist

To greet the morning with a light glow

Time: 10–30 seconds
Ingredients: Hydrosol toning mist and serum of choice
Notes: I love a hydrating mist first thing in the morning when I rise (and right before my shower) to allow all of my pores to wake up while I drink my coffee.

1. **Breathe.** Inhale through your nose and reach your arms out and up toward the sky, yoga-style. Exhale all the air out of your lungs as you slowly lower your arms down.
2. **Blend.** Put a pea-sized amount of serum into your palm and mist it twice with your toner. The combination will give the skin a dewy glow.
3. **Massage.** Warm the concoction in your hands and massage it onto your face in upward motions.
4. **Affirm.** Say an inspiring affirmation, such as, *"I feel glowing, radiant, and nourished."*

Layer Love for Moisture Radiance

Beauty is in the skin! Take care of it, oil it, clean it, scrub it, perfume it, and put on your best clothes, even if there is no special occasion, and you'll feel like a queen.

—Fatima Mernissi, a founder of Islamic feminism

When I was in high school, I never understood why my mom's complexion always looked so "wet," especially since my own skincare routine was centered around matte skin. It turns out my mom was nailing the "glass skin" look—the ultrasmooth, dewy, Korean-beauty radiance that's recently taken the beauty world by storm. The secret to this shiny, smooth-as-glass complexion? It's all about layering toners, serums, and creams and massaging them into the skin for moisture, moisture, and more moisture—with hydration levels ranging from dewy to dewiest.

One of the most frequently asked questions at the spa is, "In what order do I layer my skincare products?" Layering skincare is a lot like layering winter clothing—going from lightest to thickest consistency. (Fun fact: When we first launched, guests would come to the spa and ask this question, and I'd take a sharpie and number each product in our skincare system. This is why today you see the big numbers on the Savor Beauty bottles so that everyone can put them in numerical order to take the guesswork out!) Properly layering products means better, more-noticeable results in the long run. Massage a gentle cleanser in circular motions against the baby hair growth on your face to deeply cleanse pores. After washing the cleanser off, mist your face with a skin-perfecting toner, and layer a beauty oil and then a hydrating moisturizer on top for velvet-soft skin. Finish with an eye cream. (If you have sensitive skin, find an eye cream that has little to no scent, as fragrance can be irritating.)

A note about moisture, since hydrated skin is glowing skin: never skip the moisturizer, which should be layered on top of the serum. The right moisturizer will hydrate, replenish, and balance your skin. A rich formula should also nourish parched, dry skin. In contrast, a lighter formula can hydrate acne-prone or oily skin without clogging the pores.

I believe that our skin mirrors what's going on with us on emotional, spiritual, and physical levels. Listening to what our skin is telling us (Is it dehydrated or oily? Stressed or tired?) can help us create a customized plan for skin restoration and glow, both inside and out. And just as with our diet, our skin has different cravings in the mornings and evenings. Mornings should include a serum and moisturizer that address targeted skin issues, whether that's breakouts or uneven skin tone. And, of course, never leave home without applying sunscreen! In the evenings, our skin needs more nourishment after removing the day's dirt.

One final note, with my mom's advice about treating your skin like silk: never pull, tear, push, prod, or be harsh with the skin. Always massage, pat, and press products onto your face with the utmost loving care.

RITUAL: Layer Love for Moisture Radiance

To begin and end each day with radiant moisture

Time: 2–4 minutes

Ingredients: Toning mist, serum, moisturizer, and eye cream of choice

Notes: Remember, this act of layering love onto your

skin is a metaphor for the gentle care that we will soon apply to soul-care. See the tips on working with your skin type, which follow.

1. **Tone.** After cleansing in the morning and at night, apply a toner to prep your skin.
2. **Nourish.** Massage a pea-sized amount of a serum of your choice onto your face.
3. **Hydrate.** Layer a pearl-sized amount of a customized face cream to seal moisture into your skin.
4. **Tap.** Put a rice-sized amount of eye cream onto both fourth fingers. Dot this under both of your eyes three times and then lightly "play the piano" around your eyes to spread the cream around. This ensures that you don't pull the delicate skin as you apply the product.
5. **Appreciate.** Say an uplifting affirmation; you can write it on a sticky note and put it on your mirror to remember. For example:

"I love my glowing skin."
"I'm grateful for my radiance."
"I'm radiant, inside and out."
"I take time to nourish myself."
"I layer love onto my skin and soul."

ADVICE FOR OILY SKIN

Look for formulas with lighter oils that won't clog your pores. Watermelon-seed oil has unsaturated fatty acids that hydrate the skin and absorb quickly. In contrast, carrot-seed oil is an effective retinol to gently exfoliate the skin with vitamin A. Dermatologists in Korea always recommend increasing hydration with noncomedogenic creams to reduce inflammation that can cause pimples to form under the skin's surface. In other words, hydration can help clear skin, and if you zero in on calming ingredients, you heal versus cover up blemishes.

Don't neglect this vital hydration phase if you have oily skin, as it helps reduce inflammation under the skin's surface that can cause breakouts. You can always lighten the texture of a serum or cream with a little toning mist for better absorption, as outlined earlier in the Daily Morning Mist ritual.

ADVICE FOR NORMAL/
COMBINATION SKIN

Use products that contain ingredients like pumpkin-seed oil or rose-hip oil, which are beneficial for brightening, moisturizing, and firming the skin. Your beauty ritual should always include layering a cream over a serum to lock in moisture. Look for products that offer different formulas for different skin types for changing seasons or a morning and night cream.

ADVICE FOR LAYERING ON DRY/MATURE SKIN

Go for products with emollient ingredients like cocoa butter or raspberry oil, which offer nourishment and a collagen boost. Ingredients like CoQ10 and a natural retinol work well as a gentle exfoliator and should be applied to your skin every two to four days.

At nighttime before bed, consider doing a double layer for a boosted radiance:

Toning mist → Targeted serum → Cream → Repeat cycle

As someone with naturally parched, dry skin, I like to get ready for bed right after dinner by brushing my teeth and doing my nighttime beauty ritual. Then I remoisturize a few hours later before I get into bed, to ensure that my skin gets plenty of moisture throughout the night. One Korean dermatologist once told me that some of his clients actually set an alarm to go off in the middle of the night to hydrate the skin again! I admire the commitment, but I opt out of this midnight temptation for fear that it would disturb my peaceful beauty sleep.

Massage for Radiance

Beauty is how you feel inside, and it reflects
in your eyes. It is not something physical.
—Sophia Loren, actress

Even though I was always mesmerized by my mom's glistening skin, it was her youngest sister in Seoul who made the biggest impression on me as a teenager. She would sit down in front of her vanity table and give herself an elaborate massage using exotic skincare products, starting from her décolletage, sweeping up to her jawline, cheeks, under eyes, and forehead. She'd end with a lavish scalp massage, and when she finished, her skin was the shiniest I've ever seen. Every morning and evening for an entire summer that I was in Korea on vacation, I watched her perform this ritual on herself, which she so cherished and savored.

Today, my aunt's facial massage is the inspiration behind the Savor Beauty facials, which feature a luxurious lifting massage using carrot-, raspberry-, and pumpkin-seed oils to plump, refine, and hydrate the face. According to scientific studies, a facial massage can also improve circulation, which helps to even out your skin tone, increase healing, decrease brown spots, detoxify the skin, and reduce under-eye circles.

I love giving myself a facial massage because I feel the

soothing effects within five minutes! A facial massage can be intimidating for many people and is often viewed as a complex activity best left for the professionals. Still, once you get the hang of it and feel the relaxing results, it gets easy and pretty addictive. You can even do this as an evening ritual right in bed. And best of all, the only tools you need are beauty oils!

Beauty oils give a bit of slip to the skin, which helps with the facial massage. Even a short, sweet massage helps stimulate the skin's deeper level, which contains tiny blood vessels. This boost in circulation brightens the complexion and gives you that gorgeous radiance.

RITUAL: Radiance Facial Massage

To increase circulation, glow, and collagen

Time: 5–15 minutes

Ingredients: Beauty oil of choice

Optional Upgrades: Candle, soothing music

Notes: Here is a diagram to guide you through your evening facial massage. These techniques come from a blend of my aunt's massage and Savor Beauty's protocol. You will use your fingertips and hands for this luxurious massage following the steps listed. Traditionally, our Savor Spa aestheticians use the middle and ring fingers for more delicate areas like around the eyes, and utilize the whole hand for larger surface areas. Find which massage movements you like most and begin incorporating them into your routine.

Always begin with clean hands. Warm 5–10 drops of premium beauty oil of choice between your hands. Work in upward motions from the neck and décolletage to the head's crown. Perform each move three times with varying pressures.

a. Glide fingertips in toward the chest and out toward the shoulders, below the collarbone, and then up along the shoulders to the neck.

b. Starting at the center of the chin, stroke your fingertips along the jawline in an upward motion toward the cheekbone. This can be worked one side at a time or together.

c. Find your cheekbone and glide your fingers from the center of the face along the underside of the bone toward the top of the ears.

d. Glide your fingertips around the eyes, starting from the space between your eyebrows, along the eyebrow to the temple, and inward underneath the eyes to the nasal ridge to complete the circle.

e. In a figure-8 motion, glide your fingertips around

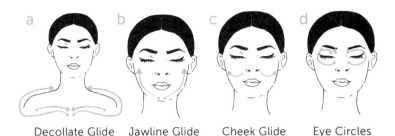

Decollate Glide   Jawline Glide   Cheek Glide   Eye Circles

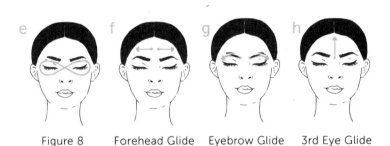

Figure 8   Forehead Glide   Eyebrow Glide   3rd Eye Glide

the eyes, starting around one eyebrow, under the eye, and crossing up onto the other eyebrow and under the eye.

f. With both thumbs, starting from the midline of the forehead, glide out toward the temple. Repeat this motion while moving up the forehead.

g. Press the inner edge of the eyebrow with your thumbs. Release and glide along the brow bone to the temples.

h. With one finger, press and release the space between

the eyebrows and then glide to the hairline. Repeat several times with both hands in a hand-over-hand motion.

Exfoliate for Renewal

We don't grow older, we grow riper.
—**Pablo Picasso, painter**

Did you know that the top layer of skin is made of dead skin cells piled up on top of each other? It's an unappealing thought, I know. But around every twenty-eight days, your skin renews itself with a fresh layer of cells. As we age—or as I like to think of it, gain years of wisdom—our skin does not renew itself as well as it did when we were young, slowing the renewal process down to around forty to forty-five days. Exfoliation, however, helps us "grow younger" by removing the top layer of dead skin cells, unclogging the pores, reducing fine lines, and improving texture. Getting rid of the layer of dead skin cells also helps beauty oils and moisturizers absorb deeper into the skin, which ultimately feeds the skin the nutrients it needs to stay vibrant and youthful.

Over the years, I've experimented with many methods of exfoliation. My first encounter came from a visit to Seoul, Korea, as a preteen. My sisters and I went with my mom and aunts to a family spa and witnessed Korean *ajummas* scrubbing naked women in every nook and cranny of their bodies. I came home, grabbed my mom's scrubby bath towel, and began abrasively exfoliating my face until it was red and splotchy. My mom caught me in the act and said, "Angie-ah! Your body is not your face! You only have one face—treat it gently. If you continue to be harsh, you will tear your skin."

My Aries nature means I always have to learn things on my own. So instead of listening to my mom, in my twenties, I loved taking out the day's stress with apricot and walnut exfoliants. As my mom warned, they exacerbated my sensitive skin. After trying a multitude of exfoliating products, I finally discovered chemical peels through my aestheticians at Savor Beauty years later. They suggested high-performance and clean peels using naturally derived enzymes and acids that dissolve dead skin cells. Unlike physical exfoliation, which uses mechanical processes to slough away dead skin cells, chemical exfoliation uses acids to reveal brighter skin more gently. The first one we launched was a delicious Pumpkin Enzyme / Lactic Acid Peel, and whenever I walk through the halls of our spas today, it literally smells like pumpkin pie baking in the oven. (I can still remember buying out the pumpkin puree from our local organic grocery store during the testing phase! To this day, we still buy this superrich ingredient from the same local grocer.)

Peels help the skin do what it naturally does, only better:

they remove the top layer of damaged skin to promote the growth of new, healthy skin, which aids in increased collagen production. Beyond that, peels are used to address a myriad of skin concerns, including hyperpigmentation (dark spots), acne, aging, and even rosacea (patches of redness.)

At the spa, we work closely with many dermatologists who refer their clients to us for facials. Dermatologist Tiffany J. Libby, MD, whose husband was one of our first spa clients in our West Village location in Manhattan, has answered many questions for our clients and the Savor Beauty team over the years. For instance, we often get asked, "What is the difference between an enzyme and acid peel?" As Dr. Libby says, enzymes are naturally occurring digestive agents from fruit that eat protein and keratin buildup. Our skin continuously sheds dead skin cells, but if they aren't removed, your beauty oils and moisturizers will sit on top of those inactive cells, and your live cells won't be able to absorb the nutrients. Enzymes help to gently dissolve dead cells so your skin can reap the benefits of your luscious creams and serums.

Acids are also derived from fruit and sometimes dairy, like lactic acid found in milk. They help soften fine lines and fade hyperpigmentation. As Dr. Libby explains, "Fruit acids react with all skin cells (dead or alive), promoting cell death and leading to forced exfoliation."

In other words, she says that they both exfoliate, but

that the major difference is that enzymes exfoliate dead skin cells, and acids accelerate the turnover of both dead and living skin cells, which makes them a better choice for more seasoned exfoliation lovers.

If you are wondering why you should exfoliate with acids and not just use physical exfoliation, it's because while physical exfoliation may give you the sensation that you're getting a "deeper" clean, chemical exfoliation with acids is what actually penetrates your skin. This removes dead skin cells to exfoliate and brighten your complexion. Many don't realize that chemical exfoliation is also much gentler on the skin than physical scrubs, which often leave skin more irritated.

Chemical exfoliation encompasses two groups of acids: AHAs (alpha hydroxy acids) and BHAs (beta hydroxy acids). Alpha hydroxy acids are a group of natural acids found in foods. Alpha hydroxy acids include citric acid (found in citrus fruits), glycolic acid (found in sugarcane), lactic acid (found in sour milk and tomato juice), malic acid (found in apples), tartaric acid (found in grapes), and others. Lactic acid, an AHA, is great for dry skin, since it's gentle and effective without stripping too many oils from the skin's surface. We chose lactic acid for our Pumpkin Enzyme Peel (the one that smells like pumpkin pie in our spas.)

For our spa guests with more oily skin types, Dr. Libby and Savor Beauty aestheticians recommend a BHA (i.e., salicylic acid), because it is oil-soluble and works deeper within the skin to remove sebum, decongest pores, and work wonders treating acne-prone skin.

RITUAL: Exfoliate for Renewal

To dissolve dull and dead skin for cellular regeneration

Time: 1–3 minutes, or as instructed on the label
Ingredients: AHA or BHA peel of choice
Optional Upgrades: Spa brush
Notes: I like to do my peels in the shower, but you can also do this during an at-home facial.

1. **Cleanse.** Wash hands and face thoroughly. You can do the double-cleanse ritual before applying the peel.
2. **Apply.** Use a mask brush or clean fingers to apply an even layer (¼ teaspoon should be enough) of the peel to cleansed skin. In Savor Beauty + Spa treatments, our aestheticians massage the peel into the skin, which I love to do in the shower.
3. **Remove.** Follow label instructions. Your skin can tingle but should never burn. Our aestheticians always ask guests, "On a scale from one to ten, ten

being the strongest, and one being the mildest, how do you rate the tingle?" Always remove the peel if the number goes above five to seven. Take the peel off thoroughly with moist cotton pads, a soft towel, or wash off with water.

4. **Tone.** Apply a balancing toner on the face to rebalance the skin's pH.

5. **Nourish.** Pat and press a pea-sized amount of a serum of your choice onto your face.

6. **Hydrate.** Layer a pearl-sized amount of a customized cream to seal the moisture in your skin.

Important Notes for Peels

- Stronger is not always better. When in doubt, always choose a lower-percent potency and slowly build up.
- Keep the application of the peel ¼ of an inch away from the eye, nostril, and lip areas.
- Do *not* apply on open wounds, freshly shaved skin, or less than twenty-four hours after dermabrasion.
- There may be some mild blushing of the skin; it should be a temporary effect of circulation.

Your Radiant Skin Plan

1. **Customize.** Commit to trying these beauty rituals and getting to know your skin. I like to cleanse, mist, and hydrate with a serum, moisturizer, and eye

cream at night (Savor Beauty's 0–5 skincare system). Every morning, I mist and hydrate after showering. Choose a brand you love; the essential thing is to take the time for self-care morning and night.

- NIGHTLY DOUBLE-CLEANSE RITUAL (to cleanse skin at night)
- DAILY MORNING MIST RITUAL (to refresh and hydrate skin)
- LAYER LOVE FOR MOISTURE RADIANCE (to get radiant moisture)
- RADIANCE FACIAL MASSAGE (to increase circulation and collagen)
- EXFOLIATE FOR RENEWAL (to increase cellular regeneration)

2. Schedule. Write in your planner or put in a GCal reminder when you will do these rituals. Remember that scheduling in rituals prioritizes *you*!

3. Cleanse. Cleanse and hydrate your skin every night while saying affirmations as a foundation for your self-love journey.

GET LIT FROM WITHIN

Y ou're glowing!" is a blush-worthy compliment that extends beyond one's complexion (which we've just learned how to revitalize in week 1) and is often associated with notable moments like being pregnant, working out, falling in love, or getting a pampering facial. Yet I believe that a lit-from-within quality also comes from living the most authentic expression of our radiant selves. When we become one with our essence, aka our soul or inner being, our inner beauty beams from our pores and radiates into every part of our lives.

Connecting to one's soul is the most important relationship goal that we will ever have. When we do this, we begin choosing authenticity over approval, which is true freedom. We thrive and bask in the beauty of alignment, confidence, clarity, and self-love. Contrary to what most people think or may try to tell you, this is not narcissism; it's the kind of love for yourself that overflows from within—an abundant, radiant light source—and enriches the lives of others, too. Once you discover and enjoy a whole relationship between you and your inner being, every other relationship falls into place. The vibrancy of our attention and curiosity burst open our joie de vivre. This ignites our radiance, and before we know it, an entire room.

"Lit-from-Within" Love

My mom's very wise words, "Treat your skin like the most expensive silk on earth," can be applied to the internal process of finding your authentic radiance. When we are soft, gentle, and kind to ourselves, we allow ourselves to be raw, intimate, and vulnerable. When I went through the journey to discover this myself, what emerged was an inner essence that felt warm and loving.

It wasn't always this way, however. There was a time when I did not like being with myself. When I was alone, there were a lot of cold, harsh thoughts: "Work harder, do better, succeed more." These voices came from my upbringing, the need for society's approval, and self-imposed judgments. I turned to career distractions to block it all out, but the more achievements and possessions I amassed, the more my inner light dulled and dimmed.

The rituals in this chapter brought my inner being back to life and have sustained my radiance and vibrancy. The secret lies in connecting to our essence every day and igniting our desires and passions. To do this in my own life, I began "dating" myself by scheduling Radiance Rituals and Radiance Retreats into my planner and treating them like real dates with a friend or lover. I also had exploration playdates with my passions, interests, and curiosities. I created, enjoyed, relished, engaged, and connected with myself in a way that I never had before. I began engaging with my surroundings and became immersed and present—breathing, savoring, and appreciating.

These moments alone were a doorway to unlocking the mysteries of my soul. They helped me to understand myself, my relationships, and the world around me. Even so, I didn't intellectualize the journey that much; I allowed myself to simply savor what I called "delicious moments"—and got out of my head and into my body. Through it all, the hardest part for this overachiever and overdoer was not pushing or trying so hard. At first, it felt like I was wasting time and being "lazy" by not constantly working and instead enjoying things like cooking and meditating. What's more, I worried about "losing my edge." If I didn't constantly work under pressure, stress, and duress, would I still be able to achieve success? But basking in the realm of play felt so good, warm, and fun that I enjoyed it more and more as time went on. There was an irresistible force that inspired me to do more to discover and be with my inner essence.

What happened next was nothing short of a miracle: over time, I went from self-loathing to self-loving. I began enjoying solitude because the inner sanctuary that I created felt nourishing and soothing. People started commenting on my "glow," "halo," and "aura"; they wanted to be around this radiant energy, and surprisingly, I now liked being around myself, too. Instead of giving to loved ones from an empty cup, I gave from one that was overflowing (we'll talk more about this in later chapters, so you can do it, too). The "lit-from-within" love that I gave myself reflected in the relationships all around me. And then that love came back full circle to me.

Oh, and those worries about losing my edge? The contrary happened: a floodgate of creativity, inspiration, and *sustainable* success opened up instead. And this time it was different. Instead of furrowed brows and struggles, there was a juicy abundance that flowed with ease and little effort. Instead of aging through the process, it was as if I'd found the *real* fountain of youth; I felt lighter and looked younger than ever.

Ready to get lit from within? Let's ignite your inner glow.

Radiance Rituals

People, even more than things, have to be restored, renewed, revived, reclaimed, and redeemed. . . .
—**Audrey Hepburn**

Imagine if we relinquished the idea of growing old with all of its negative associations of getting tired, wrinkly, and frail. And imagine if the fountain of youth could be found within yourself. I've discovered this through Radiance Rituals, the grounding practices that illuminate our inner beauty, brilliance, and balance. They're the most radical, deep, and loving care that we can actively give ourselves. When we punctuate our days with simple-yet-meaningful rituals, we express natural beauty from our soul that allows us to feel blissful and look radiant. The light of bliss imparts a glow that others notice—that attractive and charming "je ne sais quoi" quality.

Infusing our days and nights with Radiance Rituals gets us in touch with our authentic beauty and nourishes us from the inside out. It's self-restoration by way of rest, re-laxation, and rejuvenation. These rituals give us the space to dive below the skin to find our joie de vivre.

We can ritualize anything in life by infusing our days, weeks, months, and years with meaningful activities: savor-ing our morning coffee while enjoying the rich aroma and warm cup in our hands, turning the shower into a spa sanc-tuary with candles and oxygenating plants, elevating our beauty routine, practicing yoga in a sacred space, or simply watering a flower that makes us happy. It's about the energy we infuse into these routines that elevates them into Radi-ance Rituals. We can do these rituals disconnected from our spirit, or we can choose to access our radiant life force as we move through each one. The difference is in the attention and intention that we give to each endeavor, enjoying and savoring the moments.

Here's how I elevate activities from routine chores to Radiance Rituals:

1. **Affirmations:** I like to say a simple and profound statement to raise my vibration, like, *"I see bliss and beauty everywhere."*

2. **Senses:** I enjoy activating sensory experiences, whether by smelling essential oils for an aromatherapy benefit, listening to baroque music on a Sunday morning, or savoring afternoon tea and treats with friends.

3. **Space:** Creating time and a beautiful space for rituals makes it a unique experience. For example, I cleanse and hydrate my face every night before bed (time), and my bathroom has a beauty altar with my numbered Savor Beauty skincare (space), with crystals and candles.

4. **Gratitude:** I believe that what you're grateful for grows. I like to end each ritual with silent appreciation: "I am grateful for _____"; or "I appreciate _____"; or I love _____."

5. **Vibration:** Everything around us is energy, and I like to elevate my rituals with high-vibrational people (those with positive intentions and qualities you admire) and things. For example, having an

amethyst roller, which promotes serenity and calm, elevates my facial massage ritual for a neck-to-scalp massage.

RITUAL: Radiance Rituals

To connect to your soul, aka, inner being or essence

Time: 15–30 minutes

Ingredients: Journal or planner, pen and paper, or a digital device

Optional Upgrades: Candle, crystals, beauty altar, music, dim lights

Notes: Throughout the rest of the book, you will be carving out time for rituals that will raise your radiance vibration. Please take note of what resonates and begin infusing those rituals into your days, weeks, and months until they become a habit.

1. **Create.** Begin an ongoing list of Radiance Rituals you want to try and experience. You can create this in a journal, a digital device, or on a spreadsheet.

2. **Experiment.** Once a week, plan out your rituals (I like to get organized on Sundays in the *Savor Beauty Planner*). Think of this time as your commitment

to *you* and your self-love journey. Throughout the themed weeks in this book, experiment and customize the rituals to suit you. Keep the rituals that resonate with you, and try to begin and end each day with a ritual. For example:

a. Every day: A.M. and P.M. beauty rituals

b. Monday: Breath work

c. Tuesday: Face-mask ritual

d. Wednesday: Beauty smoothie

e. Thursday: Meditation ritual

f. Friday: Forest-bathing ritual

g. Saturday: Cooking

h. Sunday: Spa rituals

3. Plan. Treat these Radiance Rituals like real dates with a loved one, and make sure you have the right tools and materials in advance.

Radiance Retreats

Temporarily closed for spiritual maintenance.
—**Unknown**

I began creating Radiance Retreats after my twenty-year marriage ended—a time when my lit-from-within quality dimmed under the stress and sadness of divorce. My husband and I had evolved into friends, and I feel enormously grateful and humbled to have such a wonderful friendship, father to our daughter, and support system to this day. Even so, I ventured into the world as a single mom in New York City, feeling scared and empty. I did not know who I was outside of being a wife, mom, and business owner. Though I would show up to work wearing a mask that made others think I was strong, the reality was that in the beginning, I was crumbling inside.

For the first decade of my daughter's life, I had my little best friend next to me, and we were attached at the hip. My husband cooked dinners during that time, and we always had a family meal in the evenings. So, after our separation, when my little girl packed her bags to spend her first week at her dad's house, I was not used to being alone with a blank canvas of unfilled time. My first instinct was to head into work on a weekend or curl up in bed, feeling depressed and alone. After the first day of feeling down, however, I decided to plan activities during my "time off" that made me feel alive and vibrant. I didn't know it then, but I was learning how to find my bliss, raise my frequency, and shine on my own.

Here's an excerpt from a blog post that I wrote at the time:

> I live on the Upper West Side and always stay within a ten-block radius of my home. I have become

an introvert over the years, yet I want to learn how to cook, get over my fear of meditation, and learn to like myself. During this retreat, I have decided to step out of my comfort zone to head downtown, meet new people, throw a dinner party, learn to meditate, and contemplate self-love.

Intention: To feel good, unconditionally

Day 1: Self-Love Meditation

Meet up with a new friend to do a self-love meditation at an emotional-fitness gym (yes, that exists!) in Chelsea.

Day 2: Cook and Host a Self-Care Supper

Cook a new Korean dish recipe

Listen to inspirational podcasts

Buy lavender-colored roses

Host dinner gathering with friends

Day 3: Renew Spirit

Read *Inward* by Yung Pueblo

Go to a Korean spa to sit in a volcanic sand bath

The Magic That Emerged

- Meditation was mind-blowing, and I can do it!
- Learned how to look someone in the eye for two minutes at the emotional-fitness gym!
- Am going to a hip hop class with new friends (eeeek!).
- Love cooking, and the dish was a hit!

- Had soulful conversations with amazing people.
- Committed to walking 10K steps a day (averaging 5K steps now).
- Became a member of the emotional-fitness gym, and, yes, it's downtown!

There is a difference between Radiance Rituals and Radiance Retreats. While Radiance Rituals are small, private ceremonies and little replenishments for inside-out glow, Radiance Retreats are more significant moments to fill our well more substantively. They can consist of an afternoon outing, a one-day staycation, a weekend getaway, or a real vacation. Think of them as self-love adventures, self-care sabbaticals, exploration playdates, inspiration getaways, creativity excursions, and frequency equilibriums. They're intimate, inspired, and sensorial retreats that connect us with the most profound ways that we need to be loved. When we do enough of these Radiance Retreats, the love we give ourselves flows back into the world and into our relationships.

Our lit-from-within vibrancy comes from the quality time that we devote to being kind to ourselves; we pay attention to our inner being by nurturing and playing. Over time, the radiant source we experience during these retreats can be accessed throughout the day, bringing bliss and flow to our everyday lives, whether we are alone or with others. The following plan will get you started.

RITUAL: Radiance Retreats

To replenish your radiance

Time: Your choice!

Ingredients: Quiet space, pen and paper or a digital device

Optional Upgrades: Candle, crystals, *Savor Beauty Planner*

Notes: You can plan many of these activities for the evening, a day off, a weekend, or a vacation. You can go solo or with others—just make sure you honor your desire to replenish and renew your mind, body, and soul.

1. **List.** Create a list of adventures and getaways that you want to experience. These can be big or small, a bucket list of sorts. The only stipulation is that you should feel inspired by the retreat to awaken your spirit and give you rest and rejuvenation.

   Here's a list of the Radiance Retreats that I created for myself when I first began planning them. You will notice that some of the activities require budgeting and some are 100 percent free!

   a. Swim in Jersey Shore's ocean waves

   b. Chant during meditation

c. Visit New Hampshire

d. Do a volcanic sand bath

e. Jump off a rock and into a waterfall

f. Walk under the stars in pure darkness

g. Swim in Lake George

h. Practice yoga on a barge

i. Take a Mexican street-taco cooking class

j. Walk through Central Park

k. Dance at a picnic in Central Park

l. Attend an air show

m. Go to a drive-in movie

n. Travel to Cancun

2. Choose. Pick a date and activity from your list for your next Radiance Retreat. Highlight it in your calendar so that you will better commit to it.

3. Intend. Start with an intention before each of these retreats. How do you want to feel?

4. Plan. Begin planning logistics so that you can relax once you are on the retreat.

5. Savor. Enjoy, observe, write, reflect, and recharge!

Inner Essence

It takes courage to grow up and become who you really are.
—E. E. Cummings

One of my good friends is one of New York City's most in-demand sex and relationship therapists, who knows how to empower clients to find their "lit-from-within" self-love. We always have stimulating conversations about general topics that her clients struggle with—from thirty-something Manhattanites who have screaming biological clocks, to overworked couples who are time- and sex-deprived. One day, she told me about how she was having her own issues with a man she was dating; they were having a hard time being vulnerable with each other. I asked her if she felt that she could be intimate beyond sex with him, and, to my surprise, she paused. "Hmmm," she said. "I can solve it for my clients, but I'm not sure if I've thought about what intimacy means in my case." It was the "shoemaker always wears the worst shoes" scenario.

This conversation made me want to delve further into the topic. That night, I looked up intimacy's definition: "Deeply knowing another person and feeling deeply known."

It got me to wonder: "Do I even know myself?"

If I were to ask you, "Who are you?" chances are you would feel overwhelmed in an attempt to answer the question. Like many people, I labeled myself with multiple roles: "I am a wife. I am a mom. I am a daughter. I am a sister. I am a performer. I am a boss. I am a creator. I am a founder." However, the definition of intimacy—*feeling* deeply known—inspired me to feel who I am on the inside versus define myself through labels. I have learned that *feeling* who "I am" taps into the energetic life force that exists within the body, while *defining* who "I am" keeps us in the limited mind of the head.

In the beauty industry, a product's essence possesses a quality in abundance or concentrated form. Similarly, our inner essence is a significant element, quality, or aspect of ourselves. We are sophisticated beings with many complex layers, but we create emotional closeness or intimacy with our inner being when we connect with our essence. This essence evokes a private, warm, and cozy feeling that makes it safe for unconditional trust, care, and acceptance to come out and play. Everyone's essence is unique; mine feels like the softest fuzz and warmest love, which was the complete opposite of the hard-core businesswoman persona I'd created. In subsequent workshops, where I have done the following meditation ritual with participants, they have described their essence as "strong," "powerful," "loving," and "goddess energy." When we cultivate a relationship with our inner essence, our soul radiates its magnificence.

Eventually, "I am x, y, z" labels transform into the simple and stunning statement of "I am."

RITUAL: Inner Essence Meditation
To connect to your essence

Time: 10–15 minutes

Ingredients: Quiet space, pen and paper or a digital device, beauty oil

Optional Upgrades: Candle, crystals, beauty altar

Notes: This morning meditation ritual is what I use to allow intimacy (again, "feeling deeply known") to light up my inner essence. For me, it is a staple for inner beauty, brilliance, and balance. Just as nourishing skin pores with serums and moisturizers is essential for skin radiance, this is a daily morning ritual for soul radiance that I cannot skip. Your essence can evolve over time, just like fine red wine. Keep tuning in and staying connected.

1. **Nourish.** Apply a beauty oil to your face for deep hydration. Affirm your glow by saying, "I am glowing and radiant," or another phrase that feels empowering to you.

2. **Breathe.** Place your left hand on your heart, and

your right hand on your stomach. Do two quick inhales—one heart inhale, one stomach inhale—and then one long exhale. Repeat up to ten times.

3. **Tune.** Focus on your gut area and tune in to your essence. Allow yourself to feel without forcing anything. When you sense a vibration (the essence) in your stomach or gut area, finish this sentence: *"It feels like _____."* If it's easier, you can describe this vibration as a noun and then create adjectives to describe it. For example:

"It feels like a white puff ball. It feels warm like the sun. It feels soft. It feels loving."

4. **Distill.** Extract one or two words that describe your essence, such as "soft warmth." These words will be your affirmation for the chant in the next step. Be patient with this process; you may connect to your authentic essence the first time, or it may take you a few tries before you sense anything. Don't give up—this is important soul-care!

5. **Chant.** Keeping your left hand on your heart and your right hand on your stomach, begin breathing in and out slowly. As you breathe in, silently say, *"I am."* As you exhale, silently say your affirmation. Send that vibration out into the world, allowing your mantra to illuminate your entire body. Repeat until you can feel your body basking in the vibration of your words.

6. **Visualize.** Imagine this inner essence radiating from your pores, eyes, and voice. Remember throughout the day that you have access to this powerful resource to help you stay connected and radiant, inside and out.

Passion

Passion is energy. Feel the power that comes
from focusing on what excites you.
—Oprah Winfrey

A common question that people ask me is, "How do I find my passion? I don't know how to find what I'm passionate about." Some of us seem to be born knowing our passions, while others might spend their entire life searching. People often think that they need to think about what they are passionate about, but I believe passion is a matter of the heart, not the head. People also think that passion is something that finds them, but I define passion as our soul's *focused desire*. We invest time and energy in curiosities, interests, and explorations that pique our interests.

Discovering passion can happen gradually. The first spark is always a little interest, and this leads to paying attention, imagining, going deep, and interacting. For example, let's say you first hear about something that catches your attention (such as art, gardening, salsa dancing) in an article or from a friend. You can then attend a workshop or go to an event about this topic. Curiosity, then, may inspire you to lean in to learn more. You might try it out yourself. Your interest slowly becomes a hobby. Before you know it, it's a passion you want to share with others.

We can apply focused desire to any activity: making a banana bread, taking a class on essential oils, playing the piano, reading a book, starting a garden, or taking art lessons. Whatever you choose, go deep with what you love, and it will ignite an inner fire that engages your entire being and lights up boundless beauty in and around you.

RITUAL: Passion + Desire

To ignite passion

Time: 30+ minutes

Ingredients: Pen and paper or a digital device

Optional Upgrades: Candle, crystals, essential oil (citrus or peppermint)

Notes: Write down the answers as they come to you. You can also do this exercise with a partner who knows you well. This list will be an essential foundation to add to your Radiant Retreats.

1. **Breathe.** Close your eyes, relax your jaw, breathe in and out. Allow your belly to rise up and down, and notice your shoulders relaxing with each inhalation and exhalation. If using an essential oil, breathe in the revitalizing aroma.

2. **Ask.** Choose to answer some of the following questions to begin noticing sparks of passion.

    a. Look at your book collection, magazines, and credit-card statements. Are there any recurring themes?

    b. What subjects do you consistently gravitate toward?

    c. What do you spend your time, money, and energy on?

    d. When do you feel ignited, interested, alive?

    e. What do you love to talk about with friends and family?

    f. What do you enjoy learning about?

    g. Do you feel excitement (or perhaps even a little fear) when you think of a certain topic or possibility?

    h. What columns or TV shows do you consistently like to read or watch?

3. **Schedule.** Add items from your list to your Radiance Retreats. For example, if you love salsa dancing, sign up for a virtual or in-person class.

Commit to going deep with your passion at least once a week!

Brilliance

You are imperfect, permanently and inevitably flawed.
And you are beautiful.
—**Amy Bloom, American author**

I once commissioned an artist friend, Amy Whitman, to create a Kintsugi painting series for my dining nook. There are four paintings with different colors, ranging from midnight blue to amethyst purple, each with glistening gold dripping from the top. Kintsugi is the Japanese concept of putting broken pottery pieces back together with gold glue instead of throwing out the broken artwork. A more authentic and beautiful piece of art emerges when we recognize, embrace, and appreciate flaws and imperfections. The golden glue symbolizes radically accepting and then elevating parts of ourselves that have been ostracized, broken, or discarded.

This is where we can begin to create our own unique definitions of beauty. What makes you imperfect is also what makes you brilliant. It's an inside job to go deeper to access real, sustainable loveliness. We all have an inner judge or critic that cuts us off from our sense of beauty, love, intimacy, and wholeness. We deem parts of ourselves imperfect or broken, and we discard this expression of our true selves. Self-compassion, kindness, and self-awareness are the golden glue that holds together the cracks and chips that make us each so special and give us our lit-from-within beauty. We must acknowledge and accept all parts of who we are—the good and not-so-good aspects that are ready for growth, expansion, healing, and evolution.

We can put back together the pieces of ourselves that foster trust, care, and acceptance. We must incorporate our wounds into who we are, rather than merely burying and forgetting about them. It takes a willingness to make mistakes and to learn from them. This process helps us clarify what we like, don't like, want, don't want, value, don't value. This next ritual will help you embrace and highlight your one-of-a-kind beauty because of your cracks and imperfections.

RITUAL: Kintsugi Gold

To allow your brilliance to shine through

Time: 15–30 minutes

Ingredients: Quiet space, pen and paper or a digital device

Optional Upgrades: Candle, crystal, soothing music

1. **Breathe.** Close your eyes, breathing in and out and relaxing any tension or tightness, until you feel deeply grounded.

2. **Observe.** Is there an aspect of yourself that you are having a hard time accepting? Is there a part that feels broken? For example:

   I come across as loud and brash when I feel threatened by others.

3. **Empathize.** Sometimes the broken parts of us hold on to past hurt and need more profound healing. In this case, therapy is always helpful for processing. Sometimes the parts of us that we don't accept are part of our brilliance; for example, being loud and brash could also mean you are protecting a softer, sweeter center. Deeper understanding encourages self-intimacy, trust, and care versus harsh judgments. Consider a statement like this:

   When I feel vulnerable, I become defensive. I know I do this to protect my softer side.

4. **Appreciate.** Let's take time to acknowledge and value this part of you. Does it hold a lesson? Is this a part of you that needs acceptance, or is it a point of growth and improvement? Try to discover the more significant gift that lies beneath the surface.

Your Lit-from-Within Plan

1. **Customize.** Decide which rituals you will do this week. My suggestion is to try them all and then ritualize those that resonate.
   - RADIANCE RITUALS (to connect to your soul throughout the day)
   - RADIANCE RETREATS (to replenish your radiance and spirit)
   - INNER ESSENCE MEDITATION (to connect to your inner light)
   - PASSION + DESIRE (to ignite your inner fire)
   - KINTSUGI GOLD (to allow your brilliance to shine through)

2. **Plan.** Write in your planner or put in a GCal reminder when you will do these rituals. Remember that scheduling in rituals prioritizes *you*!

3. **Cleanse.** Don't forget to cleanse and hydrate your skin at night while saying your affirmations!

4. **Love.** Schedule Radiance Rituals and Radiance Retreats that light you up.

ILLUMINATE YOUR HIGHER SELF

After my ex-husband and I decided to amicably go our separate ways, I launched myself into the Manhattan dating world as a single mom in her forties. It was a scary and daunting move after twenty comfortable years of marriage, to then land in this unknown world of dating apps (a platform that didn't exist when I was in my twenties!). I remember going out for coffee with my childhood friend Jane and confiding in her all sorts of naive questions, like, "What are men in their forties like? Would a man even be attracted to me now?" I even whispered, "And do they expect you to put out on the first date?" With a friendly and supportive smile, Jane put it to me straight: "Angie, get on a dating app and just gauge what's out there. You don't have to be serious with anyone yet, but you will be able to start socializing again." So I downloaded the Bumble app that evening and trepidatiously began swiping left until I saw someone who caught my attention. I held my breath as I swiped right, and just like that, a connection was made. With a bit of beginner's luck, my dating life began. What was most interesting, however, is that as I treated dating like an exercise in making new friends, I actually enjoyed, savored, and relished the process of learning from new people and discovering aspects of myself that I liked—and it showed. After a few months, I noticed that men would consistently tell me, "You are glowing."

At first, I thought it was the effects of my Savor Beauty products and my skin's overall radiance that they were commenting on. But as the conversations progressed, I realized that they were talking about an *inner* glow, and it surprised me that men could sense or see it. One man drove me around Manhattan in his convertible, while sharing a story about his ex-girlfriend who owned a retail store downtown. As the COVID-19 lockdown forced her to temporarily shut down, she was so angry that she took a bat and started swinging at him and the walls. "I can't tell you what a contrast it is talking to you," he said. "Throughout this entire evening, you have not said one negative thing about how your business has suffered, even though I know you are experiencing the same business issues with the lockdown. It's so wonderful to see you light up about the positive lessons you've learned. It's been healing for me to be around you."

Then there was the doctor who told me that he felt my "pure and peaceful intentions" were very attractive. And the French businessman who saw "no bitterness, only sweetness." And the Middle Eastern man who said, "You have a halo around you. I can't explain what it is, but I am drawn to your energy aura."

I'm not a sexy bombshell (stats: five feet five, 32B), and I don't have hidden dating ninja talents. What I believe all these men were responding to is a radiant source that's nourished by *spiritual intelligence.* And this is something that *everyone* has access to. So what's spiritual intelligence? It's the ability to receive the gifts of every positive and negative situation, to have a profound sense of gratitude for what is, and to see the beauty of the higher lesson. Without spiritual intelligence, I would likely be jaded about my divorce and angry about COVID-19 having a negative impact on my business. While I'm aware of the downsides to both situations, I feel fortunate to have been married to my ex for twenty years and even more lucky to have him as my friend and co-parent for the rest of our lives. I am forever grateful that my business survived COVID-19, and we were able to thrive by pivoting and fortifying other cash-flow avenues.

I am by no means downplaying the struggles that we all go through. However, I am playing up the clarity, wisdom, and revelations that emerge during challenging times. How we see anything is everything, and this is the key to the spiritual intelligence that guides us with an exquisite sense of peace and beauty. Through this source of divinity, we can allow intuitive lessons and messages to come to us in every situation or interaction. We can own our authenticity by knowing what's right for us, not what society or others superimpose on us. We can create a vibrant, more radiant life for ourselves by sensing and respecting the universe's bigger vision and intention for our lives. We can *desire* the greater good for everyone, and along the way, discover lessons, everyday miracles, and easeful manifestations.

Ultimately, we can achieve this state of beautiful radiance by tapping in to our spiritual intelligence. It's the ability to see beyond the tangible to receive our truth, bliss, and even ecstasy, an overwhelming feeling of joyful self-transcendence. I know this may sound mystical and ethereal, but the rituals in this chapter will help you get there.

Let's start first by defining how spiritual intelligence looks and feels. On the following page you'll find some low and high spiritual-intelligence indicators.

This chapter will nurture the four aspects to unleash your spiritual intelligence: Higher Self, affirmations, intuition, and personal responsibility. We will begin by illuminating the Higher Self, your radiant source.

Your Higher Self

Challenges in life can be opportunities that
awaken a higher level of consciousness.

—**Eckhart Tolle, spiritual teacher and best-selling author**

LOW SPIRITUAL INTELLIGENCE	HIGH SPIRITUAL INTELLIGENCE
Sees problems, failures, and mistakes	Sees lessons, takeaways, deeper meaning
Finds fault	Finds beauty
Feels like the victim and blames others	Takes balanced personal responsibility
Reacts	Responds
Obsesses over details (fear-based)	Upholds bigger picture (love-based)
Not self-aware	Self-aware
Stubborn	Flexible
"I win, you lose" mentality	"Win/win" mentality
Makes same mistakes	Learns lessons
Ego-driven for selfish gain	Vessel for greater good

When I was a child, I begged my mom to "make" me an older brother. I craved someone wiser to guide, teach, and protect me. As I grew older, I found myself searching for this guiding energy in teachers, friends, intuitives, coaches, and authority figures. I searched everywhere but inside myself for the guiding light that I'd hoped another source could offer me.

When I started practicing self-love radiance, I discovered a powerful guide within me and began tuning in to my truth. I turned inward to find a wise, warm, and maternal presence that radiated healing energy. This presence was my Higher Self, or the sage "goddess" in me, and her messages were so nourishing and rejuvenating that the root of my fear, pain, and worries dissipated. I found specific times that I could easily access this well of wisdom: in the morning between the sleep and waking state, while taking a hot shower, or during meditation. In other words, when I stopped thinking and went into a deeply relaxed state, my Higher Self spoke to me.

So how do we access our Higher Selves? This presence is always here for us, and our minds and egos are the biggest blocks to this infinite source. Some access their Higher Selves through the moon, sun, a guardian angel, a divine presence, or their own intuitions. Here are some ways in which the Higher Self connects, guides, and speaks to us:

1. **Challenges and struggles:** We surrender to learn a more significant lesson that can guide us to heal and grow.
2. **Meditative states:** Our Higher Selves impart messages we need to hear when the mind and body relax.
3. **Inspirational messages:** Insight can come from messages found everywhere, such as podcasts, quotes, song lyrics, and books.
4. **Synchronistic experiences:** Synchronicity leaves us with a curious sense that we should pay

attention. Is it simply a coincidence, or is it our soul's collaborative spirit?

A deeply relaxed state is paramount to giving the Higher Self a seat within the soul. Here's a ritual to induce relaxation and access our spiritual glow.

RITUAL: Higher Self

To connect to your Higher Self

Time: 30 minutes

Ingredients: Quiet space, index cards, pen, skincare (cleanser, toner, serum, face cream)

Optional Upgrades: Candle, crystals

Notes: This ritual is an adaptation of "autogenics," a hypnotic-like relaxation technique first introduced by German psychiatrist Johannes Heinrich Schultz in 1932. I did this ritual as a professional concert pianist before each performance. It's derived from the Greek words *auto* and *genous,* which together mean "self-creation," a tribute to your Higher Self. You may want to record the meditation (step 5) beforehand.

1. **Cleanse.** Do a facial cleansing ritual with cool, refreshing water. Affirm to yourself, "I feel cleansed,

I am glowing." Pat dry and hydrate your skin with a serum and then a cream for luminosity.

2. **Breathe.** Take a seat in a comfortable position. Inhale as fully as you can and expand your lungs and belly, holding the breath for a moment. Exhale slowly. Repeat three times.

3. **Mask.** Imagine putting a relaxation mask onto your face and smoothing out all frown lines and tension wrinkles. Close your eyes, rest gently, and relax your eyes, cheeks, mouth, and jaw muscles. For five minutes, focus on all the feelings of relaxation and enjoy these sensations, letting your face fully relax.

4. **Clarify.** Think about what wisdom you would like to receive from your Higher Self. It can be an answer to a challenge, a soothing message, or anything else you need to hear today. You will be able to address this desire during the following meditation.

5. **Meditate.** Sit comfortably. Breathe in and out until you feel focused, relaxed, and clear. Allow your shoulders, neck, and jaw to release tension. Record yourself using the following script to get into a supremely relaxed state to hear from your Higher Self.

PART I

a. Start with breathing: feel your body inhale and exhale.

b. Relax.

c. Take a deep breath in and blow all of the air out of your lungs.

d. Once the lungs are empty, take a short breath in through your nose.

e. Hold the breath for three seconds, then exhale all of the air out.

f. Repeat until you feel supremely calm and relaxed.

PART II (Slowly repeat each statement three times.)

"My face feels smooth and relaxed."

"My arms and legs are warm and heavy."

"I feel supremely calm and relaxed."

"My chest feels warm."

"My heartbeat is calm and steady."

"I feel supremely calm and relaxed."

"My stomach is warm and soft."

"My forehead is cool and relaxed."

"I feel supremely calm and relaxed."

PART III

a. Imagine meeting your future self who is wise, calm, and radiant.

b. Rest until you feel a presence that is pure, loving, and beautiful.

c. Think about what wisdom you want to receive from your Higher Self.

d. It can be an answer to a challenge, a soothing message, or anything else you need to hear today.

e. When you are ready, ask for wisdom and clarity and listen.

f. Sit in front of this presence for as long as you want.

g. Be open to whatever arises: words, feelings, images, or sensations.

h. Bathe in the warm wisdom of your supreme Higher Self who is here to protect, guide, and love you.

6. Write. After you finish the meditation, begin writing on the index cards anything that came to you during this time. We will turn these messages from your Higher Self into affirmations in the following section and ritual.

The Art of Affirmations

Affirmations are simple and significant phrases frequently repeated to keep us in a spiritually intelligent, high-vibration zone with positive feelings, thoughts, and attitudes. When you are "vibing high," you attract people and experiences of the same frequency. (I'll talk more about this in week 6.) When we feel self-doubt, this sets our inner plane off-kilter. If we are not self-aware, we can begin acting on this lower vibration by sabotaging our deepest desires and intentions.

The energy behind affirmations is essential to our radiance; everything is created *first* in our inner reality before manifesting in external reality. To affirm is to assert something as real, and practicing affirmations boosts our radiance to attract people and opportunities that share your high frequency.

Affirmations have been at the core of my manifesting practices since I was in my twenties. I was broke and in debt at the time, yet I laid down the spiritual foundation for living an abundant life. I remember walking around my neighborhood of Park Slope, Brooklyn, repeatedly saying to myself, "I'm abundantly rich in all ways." It became a near-hypnotic chant, and I would say it over and over, until I could feel the vibration of these words in my bones. I believe this is why I was able to break through a lifetime of scarcity stories and am blessed today with an abundance of love, friends, and financial security.

I find that affirmations are more potent if we view them as guided messages from our Higher Selves. When we need wisdom, our Higher Selves can bring us into our radiance through an affirmation—whether it's to reset our mindsets, refresh our spirits, restore our balance, or remind us of the higher road. They are most impactful when we experience challenges and then lean into their spiritual lessons, allowing our Higher Selves to impart healing wisdom. Affirmations double as a reminder to stay in the radiance of clarity and desire versus the cloudy orbit of fear

and lack. We say affirmations throughout the day to elevate our minds and spirits.

For example, one of my friends was dating a man who
kept promising they would live together but never followed through on the agreed-upon move-in date. I encouraged her to let go of being attached to specific outcomes
and become aware of a greater vision: a shared life with
a committed partner—it could be with him or someone
else. Whenever my friend focused on what was not happening, she would go into a downward spiral. We did the
Higher Self ritual, which I'm about to share, and a powerful message came to her: focus on the general energy of
a shared life with a partner and *believe* that this powerful
vibration is working on your behalf. She created the affirmation *"A warm, committed energy surrounds me,"* which has
since shifted her mindset. Today, she and her boyfriend live
together, and she radiates the good energy of her affirmation from her soul.

Here are some rules of the road when creating your affirmations:

1. **Phrase affirmations in the present tense.**
   Putting them in the past or future creates an
   expectation with the universe that you are running
   from or chasing what you desire. For example:
   "I have boundless focus" versus *"I will have boundless
   focus."*

2. **State affirmations in the positive.** Positive statements invigorate and focus our intention, like this:

   "I am confident and focused" versus *"I am not insecure and unmotivated."*

3. **Short and simple is more effective.** It should be a clear statement that you can easily recite.

4. **Attach a feeling to your affirmation.** Stimulating your emotions will create a multisensory affirmation and convey a passionate feeling. For example:

"I feel resilient, strong, and calm. I am resilient, strong, and calm."

"I feel well-rested and peaceful. I am well-rested and peaceful."

"I feel secure and confident. I am secure and confident."

"I feel abundantly rich in all ways. I am abundantly rich in all ways."

To seal in the benefits of affirmations, I suggest the following:

1. **Repeat the affirmations out loud.** According to psychotherapist Ronald Alexander of the OpenMind Training Institute, repeating affirmations daily will reinforce positive beliefs. He suggests

practicing them in the mirror to make them more effective.

2. **Write affirmations on paper.** Writing them at least five times in a row in the first, second, and third person helps to absorb their meanings and vibrational feelings. For example, "I, Angela, feel confident and focused. Angela, you feel confident and focused. Angela feels confident and focused."

3. **Simplify your affirmations.** It is a lot easier to say affirmations when you can remember them! Try to make them as brief as possible.

4. **Listen to your affirmations to allow them to be absorbed more deeply.** Record yourself on your phone, saying them in the first, second, and third person for five minutes. You can turn on soothing music in the background and repeat the affirmations in a soft, meditative voice.

RITUAL: Affirmations Deck

To replenish your radiant source

Time: 30 minutes
Ingredients: Index cards and colorful sharpies or pens
Optional Upgrades: Uplifting music
Notes: We are going to create your customized deck

of affirmations. These are special notes from your Higher Self that you can access at any time. You can also choose one of the cards before meditation to hold the space for the affirmation.

1. **Breathe.** Close your eyes, breathing in and out until you feel connected to your inner essence.
2. **Clarify.** How do you want to feel? Here are some clarifying questions to ask yourself:
   a. How am I feeling?
   b. How do I want to feel? (If your answer to question A was a negative feeling, flip it to the opposite feeling to come up with the answer to question B.)
   "I feel stressed. I want to feel relaxed and peaceful."
3. **Ask.** Perform the Higher Self ritual in the previous section and ask for wisdom. Listen for the answers and write them down.
4. **Affirm.** Create the affirmation using the guidelines just given. Write them on your index cards. If you have an artistic hand, you can design the cards for inspiration. I like to cut and paste beautiful images from magazines or catalogs onto the back of the cards.
5. **Access.** Whenever you want guidance or want to set an intention for the day or before meditating,

refer to your deck and pull out the card or cards that speak to you. I like to take a walk and repeat an affirmation until I feel the vibration of the words in my body, which feels light and empowering.

6. **Add.** Anytime you hear, see, or receive a message that speaks to you, write it down on an index card to add it to your affirmations deck! You will add to this deck throughout the book as you discover new enlightened messages.

Intuition

Intuition is seeing with the soul.
—**Dean Koontz, American author**

I've always thought of intuition as a gut feeling I can't shake. It's the blend of emotion, hunch, wisdom, desire, sixth sense, and an inner compass. The beauty of intuition is that when we lean on and listen to it, clarity flows to us with little or no effort; it becomes one of our most powerful decision-making tools. The more we use our intuition, the more we illuminate our Higher Selves.

When I was in my twenties, my then fiancé, Marc, and I walked around Brooklyn looking for an apartment to rent. We could only afford $600 a month, so I put up one hundred posters with our phone number: PROFESSIONAL,

CLEAN, RESPONSIBLE COUPLE LOOKING FOR A ONE-BEDROOM APARTMENT FOR UP TO $600/MONTH.

Eventually, a woman named Joanna called and invited us to visit her beautiful Park Slope brownstone. We fell in love with the garden, the decorative fireplace, and the tree-lined street. She asked for our bank statements and pay stubs. When I showed her both, she gently said, "I'm sorry. . . . I don't know if you can afford this apartment." We left feeling rejected and deflated.

The next day, we were about to sign a rental agreement for another apartment that we didn't feel so good about. Coincidentally, we had to walk by Joanna's home to get to the rental office. A voice inside me said, "Stop and knock." This time, her husband, Paul, answered the door. He had just woken up from a nap and groggily invited us in. By the end of the conversation, he and Joanna said, "You two seem like such a nice couple, and you remind us of us when we were young. We are going to take a chance and let you rent our apartment."

Joanna and Paul started as our landlords, and after numerous suppers and stoop talks, became good friends who attended our wedding in France. During this time, Park Slope exploded into one of New York City's most desirable neighborhoods, and the rental market doubled. One day over dinner, Paul said, "Guys, we know we could charge you double what you are paying. But we also know you want to own a place one day, and we want to help.

Instead of paying us market rent, take the amount you would have paid us and start saving to buy your future apartment."

I still tear up when I think about the immense kindness that Paul and Joanna showed us. A year later, we were able to purchase our first home in Manhattan. In this apartment, I began making lotions and potions in my kitchen as a hobby. This hobby transformed into Savor Beauty, a company that supports not only my family and those of my employees, but many female-empowerment causes. Joanna and Paul's generosity was an incredible gift that keeps on giving. And it began because I listened to a gut feeling that told me to knock on Joanna and Paul's apartment door. Logic would have said, "They already rejected you, Angela." But intuition said, "Maybe, just maybe . . . try once more."

We don't always listen to our intuition, because it can be the smallest and quietest voice in the room. We tend to ignore it as "fluff" or "feelings" that are brushed aside. The only reason it's the quietest voice in the room, however, is because we don't access it as regularly as we should. The more you tap into your intuition, the more confident that voice will become. While intuition cannot be forced, it does need the space to be heard. The following ritual will give you the gift of time and space for your intuition to come out to play.

RITUAL: Intuition

To access your intuitive guide

Time: 15–30 minutes

Ingredients: Quiet space, pen and paper or a digital device, body cream

Optional Upgrades: Candle, crystals, beauty altar

Notes: This meditative ritual allows me to access my intuition and develop its presence within me.

1. **Nourish.** Apply a nourishing body cream to your belly and heart area. Affirm your intuitive glow by saying an affirmation like, *"I'm intuitive and wise."*

2. **Breathe.** Sit quietly, calmly, and comfortably. Breathe in and out until you feel relaxed. This brings an awareness to the breath and body, before shifting awareness to the bigger questions.

3. **Tune.** Focus on your gut area and tune in to your intuition. Allow yourself to feel without forcing anything.

4. **Ask.** Think about a decision you need to make, and ask yourself the following questions. Some

questions may or may not apply; use judgment accordingly.

   a. How do I feel, and what do I desire?

   b. Do I feel respected and valued?

   c. What are my lessons learned from the past?

   d. Am I being authentic and aligned to who I am?

   e. Does this situation/person give or take my energy?

   f. Does this feel limiting or expansive?

   g. Am I going toward an adventure or running from fear?

   h. Would I make the same choice if I had $1,000,000 in my pocket now?

   i. Is this the best next step I could take?

5. **Note.** Allow the answers to flow to you in their own time; you will know something is right for you because it feels freeing, grounding, and centering.

6. **Appreciate.** State what makes you feel grateful.

7. **Affirm.** Create an affirmation to help you remember why your decision is in alignment with your intuitive self:

"A bigger and better opportunity for my highest good is coming my way."

Personal Responsibility: Karma

My actions are my only true belongings. I cannot
escape the consequences of my actions. My actions
are the ground on which I stand.

—Thích Nhất Hạnh

The power of personal responsibility is the complete ownership of who you have been, who you are, and who you will become—a benchmark of spiritual glow and Higher-Self intelligence. Personal responsibility is an enlightening and empowering mindset that allows us to see the consequences, good and bad, of our actions and intentions. It gives us the courage and confidence to see the lessons learned and to commit to self-awareness. Personal responsibility is owning the countless decisions and choices that have led us to this very moment. Understanding that we sculpt our experiences awakens us to the power that we have as choice makers.

Personal responsibility is also about karma, a simple spiritual principle in the yoga and Buddhist traditions that states that our current reality is a culmination of our life choices, a direct expression of intention and action. Once we accept our responsibility in every circumstance, our spiritual intelligence can automatically shift to a higher plane because we see relationships and situations in a different light. I like to own my karma by understanding how I contributed to a situation and to learn from it. Every intent and action generates consequences and an energetic force that comes back in kind.

Embracing our karma gives us the soulful awareness that shifting responsibility to someone or something else cuts into our power. Without taking responsibility, we are at the mercy of the erratic whims of people and situations beyond our control, creating a cycle of victimization. We blame our parents, relationships, jobs, finances, economy, and other factors as the causes of our current reality. This "victim" or "poor me" mentality is not only toxic, it damages our spiritual intelligence because we don't learn the lessons and, as a result, we stay in a lower vibration and reality.

A good friend of mine was in an on-again, off-again relationship. No matter how much meditation, visualizing, and positive energy she put forth, there would be some relationship drama that would send her into a tailspin. She wanted to manifest a better relationship, yet she kept blaming him for her trials and tribulations. One day, we talked about how she could shift her present reality by accepting personal responsibility for her part of their dynamic and appreciating the lessons she's learned, to reverse the downward spiral.

She admitted that her career stress led to excessive drinking, which led to neglecting couple time and the erratic nature of their relationship. By owning her side, she began a healing process for herself. She empathized with her boyfriend, saw how she contributed to their issues, and forged a new, energetic path. She recognized that if she continued in this relationship or moved on to another, taking personal responsibility for her part was liberating: she ended the cycle of feeling like a victim and found a therapist to help her manage stress without alcohol.

There is nothing more freeing and cleansing than accepting personal responsibility during a conflict. It amps up your spiritual glow because you have illuminated self-awareness. This does not mean taking the blame for what is not yours. It simply means that you are aware of how you contributed to the situation at hand and own it, which is empowering. This awareness stops unconscious patterns from blocking a more mindful path for you. Even in challenging times, we can take responsibility for how we view the situation and see it as an opportunity for growth.

RITUAL: Karma Cleanse

To clear your karma

Time: 20–30 minutes

Ingredients: Pen and paper or a digital device, facial toning mist

Optional Upgrades: Candle, crystals

Notes: Do this ritual to clear up a current situation.

1. **Breathe.** Close your eyes, relax your jaw, and take a deep breath in and out. As you breathe in, allow your belly to soften and expand, and as you breathe out, draw your belly in. Notice your shoulders relaxing with each inhalation and exhalation.

2. **Mist.** Mist your face with a lavender toning mist and/or the space around you with a Palo Santo spray to clear the energy and space.

3. **Ask.** Consider the following questions. As challenging as it is, remain focused on your side and try not to blame someone or something else for a negative situation at hand. The other side has its own karma to handle; you can only deal with yours.
   a. What is the current situation?
   b. What is your personal responsibility in this circumstance?
   c. What were your true intentions or actions that led to this very moment?

4. **Appreciate.** Write down the lessons you learned and what you are grateful for.

5. **Affirm.** Create a renewed intention or statement for your elevated path. Write it in your affirmations deck.

Your Spiritual-Intelligence Plan

1. **Customize.** Decide which rituals you will do this week. My suggestion is to try them all and then ritualize those that resonate.
   - HIGHER SELF (to connect to your Higher Self)
   - AFFIRMATIONS DECK (to replenish your radiant source)
   - INTUITION (to access your intuitive guide)
   - KARMA CLEANSE (to own and clear your karmic path)
2. **Plan.** Write in your planner or put in a GCal reminder when you will do these rituals. Remember that scheduling in rituals prioritizes *you*!
3. **Cleanse.** Don't forget to cleanse and hydrate your skin at night while saying your affirmations for a soul cleanse, too.
4. **Affirm.** Create three to five affirmations. Write them on sticky notes, in your journal, or add them to your affirmations deck.
5. **Love.** Schedule a self-love activity that celebrates your radiance.

RESTORE YOUR SELF-WORTH

Self-worth is a deep knowing that we are of value. We radiate poise, confidence, and connectedness with ourselves, others, and our life. We often think we need to create self-worth through achievements or accomplishments. But here is the truth: you were born worthy, and self-worth can be restored if you have lost touch with it. All that's required is to delve inward and find what has been there since the day you were conceived. It's not about noticing what we do or accomplish every day. It's about appreciating our own beautiful blend of creativity, artistry, mysticism, sensuality, quirks, and poetry. When we choose to honor authenticity over approval, we stop resisting and begin accepting and appreciating our unique, intrinsic value.

Consider what Sakya Pandita, a Tibetan spiritual leader, once said: "Not to be cheered by praise, not to be grieved by blame, but to know thoroughly one's own virtues or powers are the characteristics of excellence." In other words, when we own our inner power and are unattached to praise or blame, we restore the beautiful balance of self-worth and self-love. A lack of self-worth stems from believing that we are not good enough, not meeting standards, not doing things "perfectly." We compare ourselves to others and seek external approval from sources, such as social media "likes," test scores, promotions, and compliments.

So how do we restore our worth? The solution is counterintuitive because we think our worth lies in accomplishments, possessions, and comparisons, but it's the opposite. Self-worth is about *being* versus doing; it's embracing the fact that we deserve (yes, I believe that it's our birthright!) to take up space and be loved and cared for by ourselves and others.

True self-worth is supremely attractive and magnetic because, as we will see from a child's perspective later in this chapter, how we treat ourselves is how others learn to treat us in turn. When we own our self-worth, we drop the need to defend, prove, or protect. We radiate our splendid beauty from a quiet and powerful inner resource that is worthy, regal, and rich beyond measure.

A Missed Note, a Missed Life

Just as we may be inclined to cover up skin imperfections with mounds of foundation, we often cover up our lack of self-worth by putting up guards and pretenses about who we are. The end result hides and inevitably suffocates that which makes us perfectly imperfect.

I used to tie my sense of self-worth to external approval that was related to how I looked, according to Korean beauty ideals and what I accomplished as a concert pianist. The Korean obsession with porcelain-perfect skin is the tip of the iceberg in a culture that is about doing and being your absolute very best. There is tremendous pressure to strive for and achieve perfection. For example, it was not uncommon for my aunts from Seoul to say to me, "Oh no! You are getting a little fat. Exercise more!" Or every time I would step off the plane from college, my mom was there to greet me—and without missing a beat, she'd say, "Your face is always too dry, Angie-ah. Here, put this on." In a flash, her hands would be in her purse, pulling out expensive creams to massage onto my stressed-out and dehydrated skin.

As a concert pianist, my self-worth depended on gaining approval from my teachers and mentors, which led to a toxic and exhausting pursuit of extreme perfectionism. I tied my self-worth to my last performance, and my confidence went up and down accordingly. Perhaps it's no coincidence, then, that the impetus to change came from one such suffocating experience.

Years ago, I was set to perform at a chamber-music festival in Europe after being mentored by my college idol, Steven Isserlis, one of the world's most accomplished cellists. He was in the audience, and all was going well, until I missed a note. When I think back, I can still feel the audience's exuberant energy in the medieval church where I was performing, and I remember the exact note that tripped me up—the low G-flat—to this day. I immediately felt my face turn bright red, and I couldn't breathe. It was one note out of a million more that I would perform in a ten-minute time frame. As a professional, I knew how to move on in the moment.

But that one note ruined how I felt about the entire performance and how I felt about myself. I couldn't sleep that night. "You're a horrible pianist," I kept thinking. "How can you miss such a simple note, especially in front of your professional idol? What does he think of you now?" That one mistake devalued the entire performance in my eyes and put my entire self-worth on the line.

On the plane home the next day, a stranger touched my arm. It was a fellow musician who had been in the audience the night before. She shared that she loved the performance so much that it brought tears to her eyes. It dawned on me that she hadn't noticed the missed note. I stopped dead in my tracks, and a realization washed over me. No one had died as a result of my mistake. Missing one note didn't cause the world to crumble. It didn't even destroy my performance the way I'd worried that it had! In reality, it was my need for approval and perfection that was causing my self-worth to crumble and collapse. I realized that I felt a need to cover up a severe lack of intrinsic value, and it held me prisoner on stage and off. Trapped and suffocated, I felt like screaming as loud as I could. I was no different from an inmate in jail, and the worst part was that I'd erected self-imposed bars. I knew that I had to find inner freedom and peace.

While this story is an extreme example of negating your self-worth, its message can be applied to the teen who struggles with acne, the professional climbing the career ladder, and the mom drowning in her multihyphenate roles. Once we break free of appearances and start living as our authentic selves, only then can we start valuing who we are as human *beings*.

Self-Worth Is Self-Love

To love oneself is the beginning of a lifelong romance.
—Oscar Wilde

One of the most important missions I have as a mother is to teach and model self-love. When my daughter, Sienna, was six years old, I handed her a mirror and asked, "Sienna, can you look into the mirror and say that you love yourself five times in a row?"

Sienna picked up the mirror and said, "I love you, my-self, Sisi," five times in a row with zero hesitation. And then she even kissed the mirror three times. Without missing a beat, she then looked at me and said, "Now you try, Mama!"

Much to her surprise, I couldn't do the exercise. I was trying to teach my daughter the concept of self-love, and yet it was something I couldn't do myself. It was a weird, awkward, and very uncomfortable moment for me. Instead, I started to laugh at myself in the mirror.

"How did you do it, Sisi?" I asked her.

"Because I just felt love."

"So, what is love to you?"

"It's life, Mama," said Sienna. Then, she was ready to move on to a new subject. *Love is life.* I couldn't believe how unintentionally wise this child's words were.

"Just one more question, honey," I implored. "Why is it important to love yourself?"

"Because if you don't love yourself, others can be mean to you," she told me. "If you love yourself, people are nice to you because they say, 'Sisi loves herself, so I have to love her, too.'" Even my young daughter instinctively knew that true self-worth comes from self-love.

To help you radiate self-worth, let's start with something we all do—look in the mirror—and change how we talk to ourselves about how we look. We'll go deeper from there.

RITUAL: See Beauty

To appreciate your beauty

Time: 30+ seconds

Ingredients: Mirror

Notes: The mirror is one of the most common places where negative self-talk begins. Negative messages about yourself do nothing to change the way you appear: they just create self-loathing and insecurity beneath the surface. How would you speak to a loved one? Let's use the same warmth and kindness toward ourselves.

1. **Look.** Take a look at yourself in the mirror. You can even do this ritual while cleansing your skin when you start or end the day.
2. **Observe.** What are you looking at and what are you saying to yourself? Become aware.
3. **Appreciate.** Replace negative self-talk by expressing gratitude for the beauty you see:

   "I am grateful for my freckles, which are cute and youthful!"
   "I am thankful for my healthy hair."
   "I appreciate my long lashes."

4. **Love.** Can you learn to love the attributes you've hated in the past? Expressing love for what is natural to you is the highest level of acceptance. For example: *"I love my nose, which allows me to breathe and smell all the yummy things."*

5. **Affirm.** Turn the statements of gratitude into affirmations, and let them be the *first* things you say to yourself whenever you look in the mirror. You can write any of these affirmations on sticky notes (or exchange notes with friends), so they're the first thing you see when you look in a mirror.

Self-Kindness

I monitor my self-talk, making sure it is supportive and uplifting for myself and others.

—Louise Hay, best-selling author and publisher

Mindful self-talk, centered around kindness, is the highest form of respect for your worthiness. The words we use in our everyday life have powerful energy, and they can make or break the relationships we have with ourselves and others.

Choosing your words wisely can be a challenge because we are often not aware of our inner dialogue's tone. First, we need to get a sense of how we talk to ourselves and then ritualize self-kindness. We often abandon ourselves when we are stressed, irritated, or feeling judged. The beauty of offering soothing comfort as soon as we hear the inner critic is that we treat ourselves with the respect we deserve.

If you're not sure what your mind chatter sounds like, pay attention to how you *feel*. For example, do you feel down if you skip a workout, sneak an extra treat, or have one too many cocktails? You can also become aware of how you speak to others during anxious moments or when you think no one is hearing you. This could be an indicator of how you talk to yourself when you are stressed out or feeling down, as well.

Start noticing when you snap at yourself, beat yourself up, or reinforce negative thoughts. Would you say the same thing in that tone to a friend? Likewise, how would it make you feel if a friend spoke to you in that same, harsh manner? By noticing, you are awakening awareness and recognizing it without judgment: a fleeting thought and no more. In such moments, ritualize self-kindness and soften your tone to find a new sense of calm and clarity.

RITUAL: Kind Self-Talk

To soften your inner critic

Time: 10 minutes

Ingredients: Pen and paper or a digital device

Optional Upgrades: Candle, crystals, beauty altar

Notes: Once you master step 1, you will become good at activating steps 2 and 3 anytime your inner critic becomes harsh or harmful.

1. **Awaken.** Let's get to know the inner-self judge and awaken awareness around your internal dialogue. Here are some questions you can ask yourself:
   - What words do you use?
   - Are there key phrases that come up over and over again?
   - What is the tone of your voice? Is it harsh, cold, or angry?
   - Does the voice remind you of anyone in your past who was critical of you?
   - Are you observing any patterns?
     For example, let's say you are breaking out. You may become aware that you jump to what others think: *"What will others think of my skin? It looks terrible, and they will all think I have horrible skin."*

2. **Soften.** Try to rephrase and soften the words from the self-critical voice, using kindness versus judgment.
   Instead of saying, *"I have horrible skin,"* you could say, *"My skin is breaking out because I ate peanuts, which give me hives. I will buy fruits instead of peanuts; I can make a better choice next time I have the munchies."*

3. **Appreciate.** Is your inner critic trying to be helpful in any way? Could you thank the critic and kindly stand up for yourself?

   You could say, *"Thank you for pointing out where I might be able to improve; I choose to use my breakouts as a reminder to eat nourishing foods so my body feels at its best."*

Forgiveness

Cry. Forgive. Learn. Move on. Let your tears water the seeds of your future happiness.
   —**Steve Maraboli, speaker and author**

Sometimes we hold on to the anger, shame, or guilt that we have toward ourselves, which can keep us from feeling that we deserve, or are worthy of, respect and self-love. This dims our radiance, without question. When we can forgive ourselves by acknowledging pain, accepting what happened, and identifying what we've learned, we're released from such self-loathing.

The Ho'oponopono (from *ho'o,* "to make," and *pono,* "right") ritual—an ancient Hawaiian practice for forgiveness, love, and reconciliation—is a beautiful and simple prayer that cleanses our relationship with ourselves and others. The mantra is: "I'm sorry, please forgive me, thank you, I love you" and reflects that we have the power to break the hold negative experiences have on us. I like to simplify it like this:

I'm sorry	I acknowledge the situation and am sorry for the part I played.
Forgive me	I lovingly release this.
Thank you	Thank you for the strength and insights I have gained.
I love you	I send love and allow myself to heal and flourish.

Before we can forgive others, we need first to forgive ourselves, and this meditative prayer can be a private ceremony to release blocks to our self-worth. Maybe you didn't stand up for yourself when you wish you would have. Maybe you self-sabotaged and regretted it. Maybe you were not honest and experienced negative consequences. We allow the forgiving energy to sink into our cells and seep through our consciousness. It's natural to resist the words and even feel self-conscious at first, but by repeating the mantra, an undeniable transformation will take place. Everyone's shift is different: it may feel like a slow melt, a gentle wave, or a lightning bolt. Whatever the experience, allow yourself to receive the amazing grace of freedom that unfolds.

RITUAL: The Ho'oponopono Mantra

To deep-cleanse for self-forgiveness

Time: 5–15 minutes
Ingredients: Private space, meditation cushion
Optional Upgrades: Candle, crystals, mirror
Notes: This ritual focuses on self-forgiveness to
replenish your self-worth. You can also use this
mantra to ask for forgiveness from others to cleanse
your relationship energy.

1. Breathe. Close your eyes, breathing in and out
   until you feel deeply grounded in the present
   moment.
2. Awaken. Ask yourself the following questions:
   * Do I need to forgive myself for anything?
   * What am I sorry for?
   * Where do I still need forgiveness?
   * What am I grateful for?
     For example, you could ask yourself for forgiveness
     if you didn't stand up for yourself: *"I'm sorry that I
     abandoned you when you needed me most."*
3. Choose. Focus on one intention at a time.
4. Repeat. Say the mantra, *"I'm sorry, please forgive me,
   thank you, I love you,"* softly to yourself, slowly, over

and over without forcing anything. Allow the words to wash over you like a gentle wave. Take as long as you need until you feel a shift within yourself.

Here are some other ways that you could practice this ritual:

- Say it out loud a few times first, and then you can repeat it silently.
- Listen to a recording of it on YouTube, which is readily available.
- Meditate on the words quietly in a state of peace and gentleness.
- Repeat the mantra out loud in front of a mirror.
- Play with the order of the phrases and see if you notice any subtle differences.

I Am Worthy

The only thing between you and big love is your belief in your worthiness of it.
—Kristin Lohr, founder of We Are Soul Sparks

I was packing my floppy hat and SPF creams for a last-minute getaway to Cancun with my partner when I got a call from John, the husband of one of my best friends.

His wife, Julie, was in the hospital with a brain aneurysm and had just undergone emergency surgery. John warned me that her mental and physical states were up and down. After I rushed to her side, she woke up and was surprisingly lucid and clear. As always, we shared secrets, hopes, and dreams with each other. I told her about my trip to Cancun and said I would postpone it to be with her. She smiled brightly. "No way, Angela," she said. "You deserve this more than anyone I know. You've worked so hard all of your life. Go and enjoy it with your man. I know you will return more inspired than ever and have so much to share with others."

I took Julie's advice and headed to Mexico. Yet, as I sat on the white sandy beach breathing in the bliss and wonderment, I began to feel guilty for having taken the trip at all. How could I be having such a fantastic time while my friend was in the hospital in pain? Why was I here, and why was she there? Then I remembered her words: "You deserve this, Angela."

How many times have we received a gift from life and not fully accepted it because we felt less than worthy or undeserving? There are seen and unseen gifts everywhere— from someone graciously opening the door, to getting an unexpected compliment, to going on vacation. Receiving these gifts from the universe feeds our self-worth, and as my friend Julie said, we share our inspiration and radiance with others. Upon returning from my vacation, I witnessed

Julie's road to recovery, and what surprised me the most was the renewed sense of self-worth she gained from healing. You will hear more about her miraculous story, which is interwoven throughout this book in the spirit of sharing her strength, radiance, and resilience.

RITUAL: "I Am Worthy" Mantra

To shift from feeling undeserving to worthy

Time: 5–10 minutes

Ingredients: Honey mask,* spa brush (optional), comfortable seat

Optional Upgrades: Candle, beauty altar, crystals, journal, and pen

Notes: Light a candle and sit comfortably at your beauty altar.

1. **Mask.** Apply your favorite nourishing honey mask (my favorite is the Savor Beauty Manuka Honey Mask) or create one in your kitchen by mixing one part raw honey and one part milk. You can

---

*Honey, like many botanical ingredients, can cause irritation or even an allergic reaction. Introduce it to your ritual with care and possibly with the guidance of a dermatologist.

apply this with clean fingers or a spa mask brush in upward motions. Leave on this luxurious mask for about five to ten minutes to allow the honey's natural humectant to draw in and retain moisture and detox the skin. Wash off with warm water and apply a hydrating beauty oil after you are finished with this ritual.

2. **Exhale.** Become aware of your breath, drawing your awareness to your shoulders, neck, and jaw. Allow each breath to release any tension until you feel focused, relaxed, and clear.

3. **Appreciate.** Write or think about all of the "gifts" you've received in the last week or so; maybe you got a compliment, someone treated you to lunch, or you took time for a luxurious bath.

4. **Meditate.** Choose one or all of the following statements to repeat softly to yourself for at least one minute:

"I am worthy."
"I have worth."
"I deserve this abundance."
"Thank you, thank you, thank you."

Inner Richness

You are valuable because you exist. Not because of what you do or what you have done, but simply because you are.
—**Max Lucado, speaker and best-selling author**

There are limitless riches within each of us, but so many of them have been buried by our personal blind spots and inability to see our inner beauty. Our confidence, radiance, and poise blossom when we fully own our intrinsic value. When we take a deep dive into the vast universe of the self, we begin to see, love, and appreciate just how worthy we are beyond societal labels.

I am a beach girl and love sitting on the sand in front of an ocean. The salty waves and their shimmering color, which I call "blue champagne," remind me of the immense abundance inside us. During our trip to Cancun, my partner and I were walking on the beach. When we stopped to marvel at the beauty of the ocean, he asked me, "What do you think the ocean is worth? What price tag would you put on this majestic beauty? Do you realize we all have this miracle inside us?" The answer, of course, is that the ocean is priceless. Our inner universe—the composite of who we are, our experiences, our uniqueness—are like the ocean, sunsets, mountains, and rivers within us. And yet we reject and undermine these

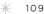

miracles. We must never devalue who we are, our innate abilities, and where our soulful desires take us. It is what helps us feel good in the skin we're in, develop illustrious careers, prioritize well-being, and magnetize loving relationships. Most of all, it keeps us aligned to the richest resource we own: our truth.

Without honoring our truth, which is an ongoing personal journey, we can fall into the trap of undermining and forgoing our truth for someone else's. I was once in a meeting with the board of a large consumer-products company that had been mentoring me for a year and was interested in investing in my company. During a meeting about an upcoming product launch, they offered advice that I instinctively felt was not aligned with the Savor Beauty brand. I expressed this, and one of the board members said, "If you don't take our advice, you will net less revenue. That's why we are where we are, and you are where you are. This is why you don't want to have investors like us because we fire CEOs like you. When we take over, that's when businesses take off. If you don't take our advice, we will know where you stand."

That's why we are where we are, and why you are where you are. These words haunted me. These men were so much more successful and powerful than I was at the time. Who was I to dismiss their advice? What did I know, compared to them? I began to doubt my abilities and value.

As I struggled with these questions, my partner said to

me, "You're forgetting the ocean inside of you. Remember that you're the one who created in your kitchen all of the creams that are in such demand. You sold the first creams. You made your first million. Without Angela, there is no Savor Beauty." It's true—and he was right. I was the one who made, packaged, and sold the products these men were commodifying, when it was just an expensive hobby. I self-funded my business by putting $60,000 on a credit card and grew it to a multimillion-dollar enterprise. I was proud of the company's mission and purpose, plus we'd survived the COVID-19 fallout with an annual profit, while keeping loyal employees who cared deeply for the brand. I accomplished all of this by turning to the ultimate board of advisors: my truth.

The next morning, I woke up and sent an email to the board members, thanking them for their advice. I decided that I would go with my own instincts on this one. Years ago, without owning my self-worth or valuing the "ocean" inside me, I would have ignored my truth and caved in to the board's demands. But this time, I took the advice as just an option, valued my inner richness, and went with what I believed. The result? We surpassed the board's predictions of net revenue.

So how does one really own self-worth? The answer is simple. Pay attention to, respect, and appreciate your unique assets, experiences, desires, and quirks. The following ritual will allow you to see how rich and worthy you are.

RITUAL: Your Blue Ocean

To feel worthy and of value

Time: 60 minutes

Ingredients: Pen and paper or a digital device

Optional Upgrades: Candle, crystals

Notes: This ritual reminds us that our inner richness is what makes us worthy, valuable, and radiant.

1. **Observe.** Begin thinking about what inner resources and assets you have. What are the characteristics that have served you well? How have you helped yourself or others? What are your natural talents, skills, quirks, desires, and other attributes? What experiences have you overcome that have helped shape who you are today?

2. **Appreciate.*** Write down each inner asset and why you are grateful for this resource or why you value it. You can also add how it makes you feel, which brings you back into your intuitive body. Say

---

*If you have a hard time finding inner qualities to appreciate, begin taking notes on meaningful compliments that you receive from others. I like to jot these down on my iPhone in the Notes app. Anytime that someone shares what they appreciate or love about you, write it down. Then go back and read it once a month, adding the ones that resonate to your appreciation list.

to yourself, *"I feel grateful for my empathy because it allows me to understand what others are going through."*

3. Affirm. Create an affirmation for when you need a reminder of your inner wealth.

The Self Gift

Treat yourself with love and respect, and you will attract people who show you love and respect.
—**Rhonda Byrne, best-selling author of** *The Secret*

During every holiday season at Savor Beauty + Spa, customers visit our spas with the intent of purchasing gifts for others. They consult with our self-care team on what they should buy for friends and family, and what always ends up happening is that they get spa gifts for themselves, too! This has become such a phenomenon that we launched our Give, Give, Get gifting program, which is now an annual tradition and extravaganza that customers look forward to every December. Whenever they purchase Savor Beauty gifts for others, we give them luxurious free gifts for themselves, like Amethyst Facial Rollers, Cinnamon Hand Wash, Caviar Eye Creams. We love to see the blissful glow we've given to our customers who think, "I deserve this!" and feel rewarded by the act of giving and getting.

After all, it's no surprise that brain researchers have found that *giving* gifts stimulates the same endorphins that kick in when we experience physical pleasure, such as eating a cookie or making love. Then there is the act of *getting* gifts, which makes us feel appreciated and seen.

Whether you're celebrating personal milestones or professional achievements, why not combine giving and getting to elevate that radiant inside-out glow? Treating ourselves to a symbolic gift is different from going all-in on an impulse buy. It can be a thoughtful present to commemorate accomplishments, celebrate a personal win or milestone, or remember a special moment. After a period of adversity, it can also be a healing gift to honor your resilient beauty.

I often buy myself a luxurious gift after I've experienced a remarkable moment in my life. I once bought myself a dress while I was on vacation because when I wore it, it felt "easy breezy," a life philosophy I've embraced. Every time I wear this dress, it's a reminder of relaxation and peace. Another time, for Valentine's Day, I bought myself a meaningful ring that I had been admiring for some time, so that I could always remind myself that my relationship with my inner being is the most important to cultivate for authentic radiance. There's something magical and empowering about wearing a piece of jewelry that has a secret meaning.

Self gifts are beautiful reminders that *you are worthy.*

RITUAL: Self Gift

To acknowledge, appreciate, and value yourself

Time: 5 minutes

Ingredients: Pen and paper or a digital device

Optional Upgrades: Candle, crystals, beauty altar

Notes: In Week 10, the chapter on abundance, I will show you how to set up a Savor Life fund to budget for splurges. You can self-gift for the holidays or anytime you reach a professional or personal milestone, or just because you want to treat yourself.

1. **Reflect.** What milestone, accomplishment, or memory are you celebrating?
2. **Choose.** What treat would symbolize this particular moment?
3. **Save.** If the gift is out of budget, consider saving up for it!
4. **Honor.** Dedicate this gift to yourself by honoring its significance.
5. **Appreciate.** Whenever you see, use, or wear this gift, express gratitude for the moment, memory, or milestone you are celebrating.

Your Self-Worth Plan

1. **Customize.** Decide which rituals you will do this week. My suggestion is to try them all and then ritualize those that resonate.
   - SEE BEAUTY (to appreciate your beauty)
   - KIND SELF-TALK (to respect yourself)
   - THE HO'OPONOPONO MANTRA (to feel forgiveness)
   - "I AM WORTHY" MANTRA (to feel deserving and worth it)
   - YOUR BLUE OCEAN (to value your inner richness)
   - SELF GIFT (to symbolize your self-worth)

2. **Plan.** Write in your planner or put in a GCal reminder when you will do these rituals. Remember that scheduling in the rituals prioritizes *you*!

3. **Cleanse.** Don't forget to cleanse and moisturize your skin at night while saying your affirmations!

4. **Affirm.** Create three to five self-worth affirmations. Write them on sticky notes, in your journal, or add them to your affirmations deck. For example:
   "I own my worth. I see my worth. I am worth it."

5. **Love.** Schedule a self-love activity that elevates your radiant self-worth.

AWAKEN YOUR
FEMININE ENERGY

Who is She? She is your power, your Feminine source.
Big Mama. The Goddess. The Great Mystery.
The Web-Weaver. The Life Force.
—**Lucy H. Pearce**, author of *Burning Woman*

'll be honest: prepandemic, I thought feminine energy was weak and passive. But I have come to realize that my underdeveloped feminine energy could actually go head-to-head with my overdeveloped masculine energy! The masculine and feminine energies have nothing to do with gender and are an essential part of every person's being. Feminine strength excels in wisdom, creativity, sensuality, and magnetism. Feminine energy also creates space and warmth, allowing us to *receive* what we desire versus conquering the big goal. Our feminine divine nourishes creativity and pleasure instead of overextending ourselves and burning out.

Let me start by explaining that when I went from being

a professional concert pianist to being an entrepreneur, my masculine energy shot up tenfold and went into overdrive. I reinvented my life from being "an artist" to becoming "a boss." I was in make-it-happen mode from dawn until midnight. NBC's *Today* show even profiled me for an "early birds" series, introducing me as a "wife, mother, and entrepreneur who runs two successful businesses. Her average day begins at 4:30 A.M." My whiplash schedule was packed with work meetings and my daughter's playdates. I was ambitious, focused, and results-oriented. Women began asking me how I "did it all," and so I developed the *Savor Beauty Planner,* a structured planning system that helps others organize what I call their "gorgeous chaos."

You will hear me talk about this whirlwind decade throughout the book, as I can't believe how long I managed to sustain that pace. In hindsight, I was falling apart from the inside out: I developed rashes, hives, chronic back pain, and anxiety attacks. My body was giving in, and I thought I needed to have a stronger mindset. In actuality, my body was screaming "STOP!" But my mind convinced me that I could and should keep going, which was a complete lie and sham.

Feminine Energy

When the 2020 pandemic hit, nothing prepared any of us for what would happen next. And as I mentioned earlier, when

New York's governor mandated all businesses to shutter for a lockdown, we temporarily closed our three Savor Beauty + Spas. My professional life as I had known it came to a screeching halt: countless press and employee meetings, QVC appearances, and spa operations all suddenly stopped. What I thought would be a two-week closure slowly stretched into multiple weeks and then months. For the first time in my life, I could not control the outcome of anything; I had no choice but to slow down. I took walks with my daughter and dog in Central Park, did online guided meditations, Kundalini yoga, cooking classes, and breath-work sessions to fill the time. I finally began listening to my body and nurturing a slower lifestyle, which harnessed the complete opposite of the masculine energy that fueled my identity.

By slowing down, I shifted from always being in "moving mountains" mode to allowing flow and fluidity. Even though my team shrank from forty to just seven people, we became tighter than ever and launched a self-love collection with ten new products in six months. We gave more to charitable causes close to our hearts, such as #blacklivesmatter and #stopasianhate initiatives. And, on a personal note, I was working less and accomplishing more. Unknowingly, I had tapped into the world of feminine energy, which was soft and receiving—not to mention as equally powerful and productive as masculine energy.

So what exactly is masculine versus feminine energy? Here's a chart to help identify the differences.

MASCULINE ENERGY	FEMININE ENERGY
Drive	Creation
Assertiveness	Connection
Protection	Warmth
Singular focus	Diffused awareness
Security	Comfort
Think	Feel
Assessment	Empathy
Goals	Inspiration
Productivity	Flowing
Conquer	Receive
Mission	Vision
Mind	Body
Solve	Allow
Rough	Soft

The masculine likes to "do." The feminine craves to "be." We all need a balance of both energies, but to compete in the male-dominated business world, I thought I had to bury my feminine energy under the masculine energy of conquering business goals. Essentially, I couldn't soften or let go of my responsibilities once I left work, which caused me to feel unbalanced, stressed, and blocked. When we put on a polished "I can do it all" mask, it creates a polarity that can affect our flow, creativity, and happiness.

The mind is the realm of our masculine energy, and the

body is the realm of our feminine energy. Our minds bombard us in the form of overthinking, crazy-making, creating stories, and ruminating. The mind may lie to us, but the body never does. Dropping into the body means leaning in to our senses to create an inner world that overflows with intuition, pleasure, and magnetism.

Here are some feminine-inspired rituals that I've integrated into my life, ones that make me feel radiant and renewed. Most of them involve living more in my body, which is about activating the five senses. When I practice them daily, I attract my desires easily and show up to work without feeling depleted or blocked. It may seem counterintuitive, but by nurturing feminine energy, we magnetize success instead of continually being in hustle-and-grind mode.

And, on a side note, nourishing your feminine energy is great for alleviating stress lines; when you are in balance, you not only sleep better, but you also *feel* better, which is the best youth elixir for tired skin cells!

Savor Cozy

Happiness consists more in small conveniences of pleasure that occur every day, than in great pieces of good fortune that happen but seldom.

—Benjamin Franklin

As a New Yorker and daughter of Korean parents, hustle and hurry are ingrained in my DNA. When I first moved to Manhattan, my childhood friend Jane (the same friend who introduced me to dating apps twenty years later) invited me to her brother's Christmas gathering. "He's getting married to a Danish woman, and we are going to hang out the entire day eating, making decorations for the tree, and catching up with friends." When I arrived, there was a spread of delicious pastries, cookies, and hot cocoa. The soft pillows and warm blankets were conducive to hours of lighthearted and unhurried conversations. Even though I didn't know anyone but Jane and her brother, I left feeling connected, happy, and fulfilled. I later learned that the essence of what I experienced is what in Danish is called *hygge* (pronounced "hoo-guh")—a cozy, content feeling that allows feminine energy to flourish.

Coming from the Korean culture, which is all about swift success and always presenting your best, the idea of languishing in cheerful comfort was foreign to me. Whether Koreans are striving to have porcelain skin, winning a music competition, or climbing a career ladder, they tend to take great pride in competing and excelling. While we can learn a lot from Korean women who give their all to beauty routines, slowing down, and prioritizing other areas of life was a refreshing concept. It helped me nurture my feminine self, fully enjoy the company of friends, and find a safe sanctuary in my home.

When I opened up our first spa in the West Village, I created a philosophy that defined the "savor" feeling. It was inspired by the unique Scandinavian concept of hygge and how I wanted people to feel when they stepped inside our world. To this day, we train our team to emanate "savor cozy" by knowing our guests' names and preferences, celebrating their birthdays, offering hot tea, and diffusing soothing aromatherapy.

Here's the Savor Beauty credo in our training manual:

> SAVOR
> relish, enjoy (to the
> full), appreciate, revel
> in, luxuriate in, bask
> in, delight in "fireplace warmth"
> with candles and family
> and friends and food,
> tucked under blankets
> on a snowy day, cup-of-tea
> conversation, scarf-
> snuggle, squiggly, warm baby love.

Women don't always make room for feminine energy, because we've been playing catch-up to the male-dominated career world. However, in the 2020 work-from-home era, I loved "savoring cozy" at home. The next ritual will give you the inspiration needed to create warmth in your environment, too.

RITUAL: Savor Cozy

To feel connected contentment

Time: 15–30 minutes

Ingredients: Pen and paper or a digital device, beauty oil or face cream

Optional Upgrades: Candle, uplifting music

Notes: This ritual will help you begin planning times to "savor cozy." If you'd like to go deeper into the hygge lifestyle, I suggest reading the book *The Little Book of Hygge* by Meik Wiking.

1. **Nourish.** Massage a nourishing beauty oil or face cream onto your face and say an affirmation, such as, *"I nourish myself and feel warmth."*

2. **Dream.** How can you create a safe, cozy space or experience whenever you crave warmth? Here's a list to inspire you, and if you can involve loved ones, all the cozier!
   - Aromatherapy candles
   - Freshly baked goods
   - Dim firefly lights
   - Soft blankets
   - Wool socks

- Green plants
- Cooking a stew that simmers all day

3. Plan. Carve out time and space to savor cozy. Sometimes getting started is the most challenging part, because you don't have the tools or time. Get everything you need in advance and make sure to carve out the time and space in your calendar. For example, if I want to cook a soup and let it simmer all day, I buy all of the ingredients the day before and put it into my planner, so that I don't schedule anything else during that time. You can also do this with a movie night by planning which movie you want to watch the day before, putting it into your calendar, and even popping popcorn to put out. Then for hygge time you can wear your softest PJs, and even give yourself a hand massage as an extra treat!

Eye Love

Dream with your eyes open.

—Alberto Villoldo, medical anthropologist and psychologist

Feminine energy craves to feel and see the beauty that's in and around us. One way that I like to access my feminine side is to play a little game of "eye love," which is about seeing and savoring beauty that makes me feel inspired and revitalized.

I love taking road trips in the car because nature's pure beauty never ceases to astound me. The pretty lakes in New Hampshire, the picturesque mountains of Vermont, the double rainbows in Hawaii, the rich sunsets in Mexico are all stunning for the eye. It's a big contrast to Manhattan, which is also one of the world's most visually seductive playgrounds. It's a city of hope, desire, electricity, and passion, and you can just as easily play eye love with the skinny skyscrapers, art-deco motifs, dramatic cultural illusions, and elegant row houses as you can on a scenic road trip. The thing is, most people don't (guilty as charged!); they walk past each of these enticements briskly, completely engulfed by work thoughts and text messaging.

Our visual surroundings can nourish feminine energy with aesthetically pleasing colors, shapes, and tones. Staying engaged with the visual beauty in our spaces and environments helps us feel happier, nurtured, and supported. Here are some ways you can bring eye love to your space:

- Paint a wall with a surprising accent color.
- Add soft and atmospheric lighting in your room.
- Buy or create a meaningful painting to hang on the wall.
- Update your wardrobe to reflect your current mood and evolving style.

- Try new makeup, like a bold red lipstick or a smoky eyeshadow.
- Take inspiring photos—print, frame, and hang them around the house.
- Play beach or forest scenes from YouTube on your TV all day long.
- Keep visually stunning books on the coffee table.
- Put fresh flowers by your bed.

We can bring nature's beauty into our personal space, too, through vibrant colors, pleasing decor, inspired artwork, stylish furniture, and textured fabrics to express who we are and to nurture our souls. The following ritual will inspire some eye love and revitalize the beauty around you.

RITUAL: Eye Love

To see the beauty that surrounds you

Time: 15–30 minutes

Ingredients: Journal and pen or a digital device, eye cream

Optional Upgrades: Candle, crystals, uplifting music

Notes: This is a ritual you can do many times as you restore and renew visual beauty around you.

1. **Revitalize.** Take an eye cream or serum and put a raindrop-sized amount on both fourth fingers. Dot the cream under your eyes three times. Lightly tap around the eyes for hydration and to stimulate the skin for healthy circulation. (Don't rub or smear the cream; the skin around the eyes is delicate!)

2. **Affirm.** Say an affirmation that opens the energetic visual field for you, such as, *"I savor beauty all around me."*

3. **Dream.** Is there any area (interior space, wardrobe, makeup, art, nature, etc.) where you want to revitalize visual beauty? Write down anything that comes to mind.

4. **Plan.** Decide how you would like to elevate your visual beauty this week. Gather tools, purchase products or ingredients, and carve out time to tap into your feminine energy's sense of sight.

5. **Renew.** Come back to this ritual once a month or whenever you feel called to it.

Nurture Touch

There is nothing stronger in this world than gentleness.

—Han Suyin, author

Touch allows us to wake up our feminine essence and stimulate oxytocin, dubbed the "love hormone." When oxytocin flows freely, it brings a delightful sense of well-being that translates into confidence and radiance. Touch also allows us to take a break from the thinking mind and get into the feeling body. One of my favorite ways to experience touch is with Abhyanga self-massage, a form of Ayurvedic massage. Here, you massage your body with warm, herb-infused oil or *sneha,* a Sanskrit word for "affection" or "love." Abhyanga nourishes the skin and soothes the body and nervous system for radiant health. Essentially, by doing this, you are enveloping yourself in soothing oils, layering them with love, and nurturing the powerful feminine energy feelings of stability, warmth, and comfort.

About a year ago, I got a painful mammogram, and a little TLC was in order. So I went to a Korean spa and discovered a "breast facial" that promised a satiny soft and smooth neck, décolletage, and breasts. If you've never been to a Korean spa, it can be a bit of a culture shock: women of all ages strut around wholly nude and completely unashamed. Korean spa culture celebrates taking care of your mind and body without stigma; self-care is a shameless, matter-of-fact necessity.

During the breast facial, the aesthetician placed a towel over my eyes, and just like a facial, she cleansed, steamed, exfoliated, masked, massaged, and moisturized from my neck down to my stomach. She soothed the entire area with warm oil, much like the Abhyanga practice. It was oddly intimate, but also not. She used compassionate maternal care that resonated with my nature of taking care of my daughter and my body. I even fell asleep because this feminine practice of getting into my body made me feel safe, allowing my mind to cease its endless chatter. The treatment was worth it; my skin was baby-soft, and my soul was soothed.

When I got home, I felt nourished, relaxed, grounded, and even more inclined toward self-acceptance. Consider how breasts are lusted after by society, tugged on by babies, squeezed into uncomfortable bras, judged by self-imposed notions, and prodded during breast examinations. I decided to incorporate a weekly practice in the shower inspired by Abhyanga self-massage and the Korean breast facial. For me, getting in touch, literally, with my breasts—with no judgment—was a meaning-ful act of self-love. Now it's your turn to try it.

RITUAL: Breast Facial

To create a satin-soft décolletage

Time: 10 minutes, recommended in the morning

Ingredients: Face and body cleanser, warm bath/ shower oil, body lotion or cream

Optional Upgrades: Clay or mud mask (a face or body mask will do), mask brush

Notes: The décolletage and chest areas are sensitive, so I prefer products that are formulated specifically for the face and body. However, you can always substitute bath/shower oil with oils from your kitchen pantry. Warm the oil by storing it in a glass or BPA-free plastic container and placing the container in a bowl of hot water for about five minutes before this ritual.

1. **Intend.** Create an intention for this practice, such as, *"I layer love onto my skin"* or *"I give myself tender loving care."*
2. **Cleanse.** While showering, massage your décolletage area in circular motions with your cleanser. Work your way up to your heart, finishing with your neck. You can also follow the double-cleanse protocol I shared in week 1, using a cleansing oil and water-based cleanser.
3. **Massage.** Using the warm oil, layer love in the spirit of Abhyanga with the oil onto your chest area. Use the palms of the hands to massage the décolletage area in sweeping upward motions toward the neck. Don't forget to reach the shoulders and back of the neck for whole-body rejuvenation. Breathe in and out, enjoying the aromas and noticing the sensations.
4. **Mask** (optional). Apply a firming clay or nourishing honey mask with your fingers or a spa mask brush

using upward motions on your neck, décolletage, and breasts. Leave on for one to three minutes, then rinse while in the shower. Enjoy your décolletage radiance!

5. **Affirm.** Express appreciation and gratitude for your breasts:

> *"Thank you so much for being part of my body.*
> *My breasts are healthy, in and out.*
> *I honor and am grateful for my beauty."*

6. **Moisturize.** When done showering, pat dry with a clean towel and apply your favorite body cream or body oil for silky-smooth hydration.

Aroma Allure

A fragrance always combines femininity and sensuality.
—**Gianfranco Ferré, Italian fashion designer**

One of my favorite ways to awaken sensuality is through smell—specifically aromatherapy. We can connect to our bodies and get out of our logical headspace by infusing sensual aroma rituals into our lives, which is a real energetically feminine activity. For example, I love to soak in a hot bath, lighting my favorite candles and putting five drops of gorgeous rose essential oil in the water for pure aroma pleasure. Since our sense of taste and smell are interconnected, I also like to savor a little treat, like a milk-chocolate caramel while sipping honey-lemon tea.

For as long as I can remember, I have been obsessed with scents. In fact, my kindergarten teacher, Mrs. Buckingham, who had become a godmother of sorts during my formative years, sent me a book she kept in a box for me. It was a book on aromatherapy, which I had read in high school; the pages were loved with highlights, note scribbles, and juice stains. Who knew that years later, I would be creating scented lotions in my kitchen? I loved breathing in their aromas and feeling transformed by each layer of perfume. To this day, I follow my nose and blend citrus, lavender, rose, jasmine, vanilla, and bergamot oils until there's a magical "je ne sais quoi" quality to the end product. When you walk into one of the Savor Spas, you might smell something like pumpkin pie or fresh lemons wafting from one of the treatment rooms. One of my favorite compliments from our Savor Spa guests is, "I love how everything smelled during my facial!"

A fragrance provokes a vast array of feelings, from relaxation to vibrancy to desire. Studies show that scent is so powerful that it plays a significant role in stimulating attraction between two people. While science links our scent to romantic arousal, I like to think that aromas keep me turned on to life by adding a sensual dimension to everyday norms. I love smelling books, candles, flowers, a home-cooked meal, banana bread in the oven, fresh coffee grinds, and perfume. I'm riveted to the present while powerful memories from the past are evoked.

So let's start bringing the alluring power of scent into your life with something we all do daily: the shower. Here's a simple ritual to transform the mundane shower into an instant spa sanctuary to tune in to your feminine divine energy.

RITUAL: Create a Spa Sanctuary
To feel vibrant and alive

Time: 5 minutes

Ingredients: Essential oils, shower

Notes: Essential oils can instantly transform a shower into a spa sanctuary. I love lavender for its calming benefits, peppermint for invigoration, and eucalyptus to clear my sinuses.

1. **Breath.** Breathe in and out through the nose during this ritual.
2. **Drop.** Put 3–7 drops of the essential oil onto the shower floor. The hot water and steam will help the oil vapors diffuse into the air.
3. **Inhale.** Savor the scented steam for relaxing aromatherapy that lasts far beyond the shower. I like

to bend from the hips and breathe in and out for an aromatherapeutic stretch!

4. Affirm. Set an intention for your day.

Here are other ways to infuse the power of essential oils into your daily life:

- Put essential oils in an aroma diffuser.
- Mist your sheets with a lavender-scented linen spray for a calming aromatherapy.
- Place 1–3 drops of citrus essential oil onto your counters before wiping for an uplifting boost.

Sound Soak

Music expresses that which cannot be put into words.
—Victor Hugo, French poet

I love to sit and listen to a waterfall as much as I enjoy the sound of laughter. As a retired pianist, music is a part of my everyday life and helps me to access feminine energy by making me want to move, dance, feel, cry, and chill.

I'm continually adding to my Spotify playlists for different moods: "Monday Morning Motivation," to "Self-Love Sunday," to "High Vibes," to "Dance Party" to "Girlfriend Gatherings." Hearing the rhythm, melodies, and lyrics of different genres—jazz, classical, blues, rock, and ballads—can move you in a way that none of the other senses can. A gathering with the right music vibe brings color and emotion to the atmosphere. This instant mood-booster adds a pleasurable dimension that anchors you in the present and helps create memorable moments.

Another way to incorporate sound is through singing, chanting, mantras, and sound baths. I first discovered sound bathing through Melanie, our West Village spa manager. We were planning a special New Moon Visioning event with self-care stations, palm readings, visioning experts, goody bags, lavender milk masks, and moon cocktails. During the planning stages, she suggested, "How about we do a sound bath for the party guests?" I wasn't sure what that was, but it sounded so luxurious and mysterious that I was game. As Melanie explained it, "A sound bath is like a relaxing bath for your spirit and soul. We can get crystal or Tibetan singing bowls (the size of a small to large salad bowl) with a gong, and it creates this soothing, echoing sound for healing vibrations. For the event, we could create a self-care station for guided meditation and a sound bath to help guests block mind chatter and connect with their bodies."

I was riveted. The next day, I googled "sound bath rituals." To my delight, I found Katherine Hamer, founder of the Singing Bowl & Sound Institute of New York, just blocks away from my home on the Upper West Side. I booked a session and walked into an intimate room with four spots set up for attendees with mats, pillows, and blankets. As we laid in Savasana (a yoga pose in which you lie on your back), she began leading us through a meditation. When I heard the first gong, I was in ecstasy. As someone who has a hard time meditating, this was the perfect way for me to get into the most meditative and restorative state. She rang up to ten bowls, each creating a different frequency that produced deep, overlapping vibrations.

Katherine explained that Tibetan singing bowls have been used for their therapeutic effects for thousands of years. I loved the session so much that I asked if she sold any of the bowls. We talked through the feeling and frequency that resonated with me, and Katherine said to come back next week—she would have the perfect singing bowl for me made in the eleventh century by monks! I picked it up on the day of our Savor Beauty New Moon Visioning event and brought it straight to Melanie, who exclaimed, "I never believed that when I suggested a sound bath that I would be gonging a Tibetan bowl made in the eleventh century!"

Here's a meditation ritual that incorporates mesmerizing sound using a sound bowl, to drop into your body and awaken your feminine energy. And don't worry if you don't have a sound bowl; that's what Spotify and YouTube are for!

RITUAL: Sound-Bath Ritual

To get into a restorative state

Time: 5 minutes

Ingredients: Sound bowl and gong, or find one to listen to on Spotify or YouTube

Notes: Try to immerse yourself in the vibration, timbre, and energy as you bathe in the sound to restore and reawaken your feminine spirit and soul. You can find a sound bowl online or at a specialty store.

1. **Breathe.** Inhale and exhale gently through your nose for five cycles.
2. **Intend.** Set an intention for this practice.
3. **Gong.** With a relaxed but firm grip, gently strike the bowl with your gong.
4. **Immerse.** Allow the vibration and resonance of the sound to envelop you, like a bath for the soul.
5. **Listen.** Follow the sound as it dissipates into the air. You will be surprised by how long it lingers, like perfume.

Soften to Receive

One of the most powerful lessons I learned about the feminine divine was being open to receiving versus pushing for specific outcomes. When I shift from aiming to get results to allowing and receiving, I slow down, soften the edges, listen more intently, and receive abundantly. I become aware of the nourishing energies around me that are ripe with gifts, insights, and lessons.

This receiving process reminds me of how the pores of our skin receive so much more nourishment when they are cleansed and prepped for absorption. In a Savor Beauty facial, we use different techniques, such as a hot, moist towel or steam to soften pores before applying a nourishing or detoxifying mask. This process melts the debris to a butterlike consistency, so that the skin extracts more easily and drinks up the mask's nutrients.

The same process occurs energetically when we prep our "inner pores," aka the soul. We soften the edges to absorb and soak in the good frequencies that are trying to nourish us. This allows us to melt the barriers that prevent the manifestations of feel-good thoughts, pleasurable experiences, connected relationships, financial abundance, and the feminine divine.

The following ritual is a meditation to use whenever you overthink the future, struggle with the present, feel insecure, or try to control outcomes—top culprits to suppressing your feminine divine. It energetically opens you up, melts blockages, and replenishes nourishment. You will shift from thinking to feeling, from pushing to allowing, and from wanting to receiving.

RITUAL: "I Receive" Meditation

To connect to your radiance and attract similar frequency

Time: 10–20 minutes

Ingredients: Comfortable seat, quiet and safe environment

Optional Upgrades: Beauty oil or face cream, candle, crystals, journal, and pen

Notes: Record yourself saying the meditation in step 4 in advance so that you can close your eyes to feel transported. Feel free to keep the meditation as is or customize the words for deeper resonance.

1. Light. Set the visual environment with a soothing candle.

2. Nourish. Apply your beauty oil (or a cream for hydration and nourishment) onto your face and affirm your glowing skin by saying, *"I feel radiance."*

3. Breathe. Take a long, deep breath in through your nose. Exhale through your nose one to two counts longer than your inhale. Repeat for a few cycles until you feel grounded.

4. Receive. Read or listen to a recording of yourself reading the following meditation.

"I am ready to receive
My vibration is open
My aura is soft
I receive and am radiant.

I love this adventure
I love who I am
I love where I am
I receive and feel radiant.

I love where I've been
I love where I'm going
I love how life is unfolding
I receive beautiful radiance.

Even when things don't go my way
Even when things do go my way
I surrender to both
I receive and feel gorgeous radiance.

Manifesting always starts with a feeling
Then it's a seed of potential
And finally, a blossomed flower
I receive loving radiance.

I savor the beauty of this flower
I savor the beauty of what is
I savor the beauty of the lessons
I receive the beauty of my radiance.

My radiance nourishes
My radiance glows
My radiance loves
I receive the vitality of my radiance.

I feel
I believe
I receive . . .
Loving radiance."

Your Radiant Vibration Plan

1. Customize. Decide which rituals you will do this week. My suggestion is to try them all and then choose those that resonate. Commit to doing them at least three times this week.

   - SAVOR COZY (to feel connected contentment)
   - EYE LOVE (to see beauty)

- BREAST FACIAL (to nourish and feel self-acceptance)
- CREATE A SPA SANCTUARY (to feel vibrant and alive)
- SOUND-BATH RITUAL (to get into a restorative state)
- "I RECEIVE" MEDITATION (to connect to your radiance)

2. Record. On your phone, record the "I Receive" meditation, so that you can listen and feel transported.

3. Schedule. Write in your planner or put in a GCal reminder when you will do these rituals. Remember that scheduling in rituals prioritizes *you*!

4. Cleanse. And don't forget to cleanse and hydrate your skin at night while saying your affirmations!

5. Affirm. Create three to five self-worth affirmations. Write them on sticky notes, in your journal, or add to your affirmations deck.

6. Love. Schedule a self-love activity that elevates your radiant vibration.

Week 6

NOURISH YOUR RADIANCE

We all know someone who radiates beauty, vibrancy, and an enviable ease that emanates a lit-from-within quality. So what exactly is this irresistible magnetism and energetic vibration that I call your gorgeous radiance, and how can you develop it within yourself?

As I mentioned in week 1, in ancient Korean times, the outer body and spirit were considered to be one. In fact, your inner well-being and wealth were said to live in your heart and to be reflected in your appearance. In other words, if you were feeling down or stagnant, it would show up in how you looked. And by the same token, a beautiful glow is said to be the illumination of your most authentic inner beauty and brilliance that shines from every aspect of your being: from your skin, eyes, smile, actions, the way you live, who you are, and *how* you are.

Because this inner essence, your radiant source, is so powerful and authentic, it creates a magnetic field, known as your aura or vibration. When you are "vibing high," your radiance erupts through the skin and attracts people and experiences of the same frequency. Others can't help but feel irresistibly drawn to the vibrant energy that you radiate. It's beautiful, it's magical, and it's authentically you and yours. Conversely, if we are emanating what I call a dull vibration, we emit an energy from a cloudy orbit, which can attract undesired situations, toxic people, and negative feelings. This is why nourishing our radiant source is one of the most significant actions we need to take *every single day.*

I intentionally placed this vibration chapter *before* the one in which I'll share my very best manifesting secrets, because of my personal experience with both subjects. In the past, I was always able to manifest most of what I desired at any cost, yet always felt empty and burnt out as a result. I was never happy about what came to fruition, because I was tuning in to the dull vibrations of fear and lack, versus the radiant vibrations of joy and abundance. For instance, my lifelong dream was to own an apartment in Manhattan and build a successful multimillion-dollar beauty business. Both came to be, but I couldn't enjoy the fruits of my labor because my mindset wasn't attuned to the right vibration. To the outside world, my life looked glamorous and successful, but I was working thirteen-hour days, and everything I did to feed my abundance felt depleting rather than restorative. Sheer determination always won me the prize, but by the time the desired manifestation was achieved, I was too exhausted to savor the success.

The Self-Love Vibration

It was only when I embarked on a journey to discover and practice self-love that I learned the importance of starting from an intentional place where I choose how I want to *feel*. The subsequent transformation is so simple yet simultaneously astounding: I allow my radiance to flow, so I can be a magnet for gorgeous experiences, relationships, and a rich abundance that I never thought possible—and it has come to me effortlessly and joyfully as a result. I'm not saying that I don't embrace a work ethic. A work ethic is an important part of manifesting. But manifesting starts with your radiant vibration, followed by momentum, flow, creativity, passion, and inspiration.

I know the process sounds like magic, but it really starts with a choice—*your* choice. There is a replenishable source inside all of us where we connect to our inner essence, infinite abundance, and juicy bliss to radiate our authentic inner and outer beauty. This wellspring within you is the richest asset you own, and it's the highest expression of self-love when we continually nourish and connect to this radiant source. Best of all, it's free and always available to you. Let's get started.

Feel Good

Elevating from a dull vibration to one of radiance is a daily commitment to the practice of feeling good, *unconditionally.* This means that regardless of external conditions—positive or negative—we aim to stay balanced and lit from within. This is no easy feat, and the rituals in this chapter will help you fluidly replenish your radiance.

According to Dr. Candace Pert, neuroscientist and author of *Molecules of Emotion: The Science Behind Mind-Body Medicine*, emotion molecules change the chemistry and electricity of every cell in both our bodies and minds. Feelings, she finds, can alter the electrical frequencies in our bodies; and as our individual cells carry an electrical charge, so does the body. Like an electromagnet, Dr. Pert says that people have positive and negative charges. "We're vibrating like a tuning fork—we send out a vibration to other people," Dr. Pert notes. "We broadcast and receive. Thus the emotions orchestrate the interactions among all our organs and systems to control that. So we're actually sending out various electrical signals—vibrations."

Throughout the rituals in this chapter, you will be asked to uncover how you feel and to identify a desired positive feeling state. Sometimes it's hard to figure out how you truly feel, because emotions can be overwhelming. One helpful tool is the "feeling wheel" developed by various organizations and psychologists. As an example, if you google the Junto Emotion Wheel, you will see that it identifies six core emotions in the innermost ring: love, joy, surprise, sadness, anger, and fear. The outer two rings drill down into more specific emotions related to the core emotions.

In order to access your radiant vibration, it's helpful to identify how you currently feel and then pinpoint how you *prefer* to feel. You can find the negative emotion that you're feeling on the wheel and look at the opposite side for your goal emotion. For example, if you're feeling sadness, look across the wheel at the opposite emotion, which is love, as a guide to get back into a positive mood state.

I have created a simplified chart, which can be found on the next page, to help you identify dull versus radiant vibrations.

Awaken Awareness

I never lose. I either win or learn.
—Nelson Mandela

Your skin and soul have a lot in common. When it comes to skincare, it's best to focus on *root causes* versus temporary solutions to skin conditions. This means being aware of saboteurs that can lead to irritations and breakouts. For example, certain foods like chocolate or cheese are common skin irritations. We can try to detox the skin with cleansers and

DULL VIBRATIONS	RADIANT VIBRATIONS
Stuck	Flowing
Reactive	Responsive
Fatigued	Energetic
Self-centered	Self-aware
Apathetic	Empathetic
Bored	Creative
Jealous	Abundant
Indifferent	Forgiving
Unforgiving	Forgiveness
Depressed	Hopeful
Directionless	Inspired
Needy	Resourceful
Unappreciative	Appreciative
Undisciplined	Disciplined
Unfit	Fit
Self-sabotaging	Self-supporting
Selfish	Generous
Irritable	Patient
Attached	Unattached
Non-insightful	Insightful
Toxic	Uplifted
Distracted	Focused
Dishonest	Honest

masks all day, but if we keep eating these aggravating foods, we sabotage any efforts for clear, bright skin. Discovering the root cause of what keeps us from having beautiful skin increases awareness, and therefore, true transformation. A very similar principle applies to many soul irritants, too: if we are unaware of the external root factors that activate negative feelings and dull vibrations, then we can easily spin out of control. This creates a domino effect, which in turn affects the vibrational frequency that we emit and the experiences we magnetize. A negative activation can come from conversations, interactions, sights, sounds, you name it. Internally, we react to these specific external conditions when thoughts turn into emotions, and, according to neuroscientist Jill Bolte Taylor, when we let the emotion soak in, it turns into a feeling within ninety seconds.

Our natural instinct is to push these negative feelings down so that we don't have to deal with them. However, suppressing or ignoring how we feel is not the answer; upsetting feelings don't simply dissolve, because eventually, if they're not dealt with, we emanate dull vibrations, which dim our radiance. This impacts how we speak to ourselves, relate to others, and show up in the world.

It's natural to react to external conditions, so how do we stop them from sabotaging our best intentions and radiant vibration? The answer is to awaken awareness, which is the first step to letting go of what holds us back. We can't change what we aren't even aware of, right? The beauty of awareness is that it illuminates the thoughts that we have—the ones that ultimately create an emotion-feeling loop and become your dominant "vibe."

The following ritual creates space for external conditions and emotions by bringing them to light and helping you move through them. Think of it like a cleanse for your radiant vibration.

RITUAL: Vibrational Deep Cleanse

To shift from a dim to radiant vibration

Time: 30 minutes

Ingredients: Pen and paper or any other method to record your answers, cleansers (preferably a double-cleanse system)

Optional Upgrades: Candle, crystals

Notes: The questions in step 2 always awaken awareness for me whenever I feel down. Fill in the blanks or write the answers as they come to you. Come back to this ritual whenever you want a vibrational deep cleanse. You may want to keep a record of your answers to see how you evolve over time.

1. **Purify.** As a symbolic opening, wash your face using the Korean-beauty double-cleanse technique you learned in week 1, "Start with Your Skin." Feel the purification of your pores as you gently

treat your skin like the most expensive silk in the world.

2. **Reflect.** First, observe the external condition and your reaction to it, with the intention of awakening awareness. This is a powerful precursor to transformation. Here is a vibration-cleansing protocol that will gently encourage you to process and move through negative emotions.

a. **I'm feeling _____.**

If it's hard to identify a feeling, you can ask yourself if there's an action you feel like taking. If you can identify an action that you want to take, this can sometimes reveal the underlying feeling. For example, if you feel like hitting a pillow, you may identify feeling angry, frustrated, or stressed.

b. **What external condition or thought caused this feeling?**

Try to be as specific as possible when identifying what the external condition is.

c. **Why did it affect you?**

Often, the first answer to "Why?" is the external circumstance(s) that led to how you are feeling. Keep asking yourself "Why?" and peel back the layers until you get to the root cause. If you feel blocked, don't judge it, and continue on. The answers may come to you later.

d. **Is there any other aspect (positive or negative) of the external condition that provides insight?**

Sometimes we focus on the negatives and forget there are also positive aspects. Adding context provides a fuller and more objective picture.

e. **Are there any takeaways, clarifications, or lessons?**

Pay attention to the learning gifts from this experience. When you learn, you win.

f. **Is there anything you are grateful for?**

Gratitude and appreciation are healing balms for the soul.

g. **Can you identify how you want to feel now?**

I want to feel _____; or I feel _____.

h. **State the following:** *"I release 'what is' and focus on feeling good, unconditionally. I tune in to feeling _____ [insert desired feeling]."*

Meditate on this statement and the vibration of the desired feeling state. Begin to notice your radiant vibration rise as you focus on this feeling.

3. **Radiate.** Create an empowering affirmation, such as, *"I tune in to feeling good unconditionally,"* to say to

yourself whenever the same external condition sneaks up on you. As we learned in week 3, in the section called "The Art of Affirmations," this is a soothing and succinct message from your Higher Self to help you vibrate your authentic radiance. Make sure to add the affirmation to your affirmations deck!

Let It Be

Let go or be dragged.
—Zen proverb

Has anyone ever told you, "Just let it go"? For those of us who tend to overthink, "letting go" is not easy and can feel frustrating. It's a natural reaction to hold on to the emotions of fear, hurt, and control, which is like dead weight that dampens our mood and dulls our vibrancy. Whether we're attached to the past or anxious about the future, a tight grip robs us of vital energy.

So what does letting go mean, and how do you do it? Something that helped me with this lesson was a mindset shift: *To let go, is to let it be.* The idea of "let it be" is to not control or change an external condition; it's important to let fear and hurt melt away and clear an internal space for a more radiant vibration. It's not about ignoring what's there; it's about appreciating the beauty of what is (the gifts, the lessons), but also choosing to focus on a new feeling. We can even learn about letting go from the natural rhythm of our skin, which is constantly turning over dead, damaged skin cells in a fascinating process that scientists call "desquamation." When a new "daughter" skin cell is born at the deeper level, it progresses upward, allowing the older cellular layer to slough off. Shedding this buildup of the past stimulates cellular regeneration and helps nutrients absorb deeper into the skin, which improves its radiant vibrancy.

Our souls aren't so different. We must allow the past to fall off in order for a renewed vibration to emerge. We don't often take the time to symbolically let go of the past. We tend to ignore it or hold on to "what was" because we've become accustomed to the tight grip. I find that letting go, releasing, and melting away emotional buildup in the face first, followed by the soul, is deeply restorative. With forty-two muscles above our neck, our faces work exceptionally hard: we express happiness, anger, sadness, joy—and we do all of this by laughing, crying, smiling, frowning, and furrowing. Over time, the internal tension shows externally through sagging skin, tired eyes, and an asymmetric face.

While letting go of whatever lowers our radiant vibration can be hard, this facial rolling ritual will help you release unnecessary gunk from the past to help renew your skin and soul, both consciously and mindfully. Facial rolling is a technique that can melt away the emotional tension we hold and let go of the skin's and soul's toxins for inner-outer radiance. Let's get rolling!

RITUAL: Self-Love Roll + Glow

To let go of emotional tension

Time: 5–30 minutes

Ingredients: Facial roller (available at your local spa or savorbeauty.com), beauty oil of your choice, mirror

Optional Upgrades: Soothing music, candle, journal

Notes: If you don't have a roller, simply use clean hands for this ritual. Close your eyes and pay attention to any tension in the face or neck areas. Begin rolling, using the following method:

1. **Breathe.** Take a deep breath in and out.
2. **Dedicate.** Is there anything that you want to let go of? You can "let it be" and melt away and shed what no longer serves you: the tight grip, the fear, the expectations.

FOREHEAD: Start at brows and roll in upward motions toward hair line.

JAW + CHEEKS: Start at jaw and roll in upward motions toward cheeks.

CHIN: Start in the middle and roll out toward the right and left.

EYES: With smaller roller, start at inner corners under eyes, rolling outward.

NECK: Start at collarbone, roll in upward motions toward jaw.

3. **Roll.** Follow this protocol, and use clean hands if you don't have a roller.

   a. Apply one drop of a beauty oil onto your forehead.

   b. Take the small end of the roller or your fingertips and massage in upward motions on the forehead. Breathe in and breathe out, asking what the tension is trying to tell you. Let it go as you relax.

   c. Massage the rest of the forehead with the large end of the roller or your palms.

   d. Apply another 1 to 2 drops of the oil onto the cheek and chin area and roll, using the large end, in an upward and outward motion. Breathe in and breathe out, asking what the tension is trying to tell you. Let it go as you relax.

e. Use the small end to massage around the eyes to increase circulation and decrease puffiness.

f. Apply another 1 to 2 drops of the oil onto the neck and décolletage area and roll, using the large end in an upward motion. Breathe in and breathe out, asking what the tension is trying to tell you. Let it go as you relax.

g. Continue the process of rolling down your neck to stimulate the lymphatic system for deeper cleansing.

4. Affirm. Write down any revelations or messages you had during the process. If there was an affirmation or message that emerged, add it to your affirmations deck.

Surrender to a Soul Collaboration

One of the top reasons that our radiant vibration becomes dull and dim is that we're always trying to control outcomes so that we don't have to face worst-case scenarios. In fact, we are hardwired to ask ourselves, "What if x, y, z happens or goes wrong?" Coming up with solutions to these imagined scenarios can be helpful and even save us from undesired outcomes, but as you will see, we often spend too much time in our heads and not enough time in our bodies.

We then become disconnected from our spirit and cut off from our energetic flow.

Sometimes "what ifs" come from deeper childhood pain. Laura Forbes, a Neuro-Linguistic Programming (NLP) practitioner, advises us to lean into our body's wisdom to understand emotional messages in order to surrender to "what ifs." She suggests closing the eyes, scanning the body for pain, and paying attention to whether the sensations are related to deeper emotional memories stored in the body. She says, "Ask the pain how old it is. As a child, what did you need to hear or feel that you didn't get at that time? And then notice that you can give yourself those things now. This will enable you to integrate those parts of yourself back to the whole."

When the coronavirus pandemic forced me to shut down my Savor Beauty + Spas and sent us all into quarantine, I did what came most naturally to me: I resisted "doing nothing" and came up with plans for all of the "what ifs." As two weeks turned into two months and more, I had no choice but to relinquish control and surrender to a power greater than myself.

I was not the only one who had a business negatively affected by the pandemic, of course, as a devastating number of small businesses around the globe were forced to shutter in the six-month period after the initial outbreak. One of my dear friends, a powerhouse CEO who had built a two-decades-old flourishing gourmet food business, said to me on a video call, "My bank account has drained from seven figures to three digits in a matter of months. For the first time in my life, I don't know what to do. What if I lose everything and have to close?"

We sat in silence. Then I said to her quietly, "What if you simply surrendered?"

She looked at me with a surprised expression. We always gave each other sound and strategic business advice, and this was completely the opposite of aiming toward a specific outcome. I thought she would resist this notion, so her response surprised me even more: "I want to surrender. Can you show me how?"

"Let's be okay with the worst-case scenario, as scary as it is," I said. "Even if you lost your business, you would still have your health, beautiful family, and all the love in the world from your friends. Let's surrender *everything* and also leave room for a miracle that may unfold."

We did the following ritual together, and she surrendered to whatever might happen next. When we got off the phone, I felt she was *truly* okay with any outcome. The following morning, she texted me. An investor had come through, and she would be okay for the next six months. Coincidence? Maybe, but these are the kinds of miracles, or "soul collaborations," that happen when we surrender to something greater than us. Perhaps the greatest miracle of all is becoming unattached to the "what ifs" and knowing that you are okay *no matter what.*

RITUAL: "I Surrender" Meditation

To let go of "what if" fear and leave room for a miracle

Time: 20 minutes

Ingredients: Comfortable seat, quiet environment

Optional Upgrades: Candle, crystals, body cream or oil

Notes: This ritual has been divided into two parts, which you can do together or apart. Replace the bolded words in the meditation with ones that resonate with you. Then read or record yourself saying this meditation so that you can close your eyes to be transported to a peaceful place within your soul.

1. **Breathe.** Close your eyes, breathing in and out until you feel deeply grounded.

Part I: Body Wisdom

a. **Scan.** Observe the body for pain.

b. **Nourish.** If you wish to use a body cream or oil, gently massage the area of focus.

c. **Feel.** Pay attention to sensations that are related to emotional memories stored in the body.

d. **Awaken.** Once you identify the specific area, imagine the body part being able to breathe in and out.

   e. **Allow.** Ask the body pain the following questions, allowing answers to flow to you:

- How old do you feel?
- What are the sensations?
- Are there any memories associated with the pain?
- What do you need to hear to feel better now?

   f. **Write.** Take note of any insights that come to light.

Part II: Surrender Meditation

   a. **Meditate.** Read or listen to a recording of yourself saying the following meditation. Without forcing anything, allow the energy of this meditation to absorb into your body. With consistent practice, you will eventually feel yourself surrendering. Customize the meditation by replacing the bolded words with ones that resonate, such as "abundance" or "peace."

I SURRENDER.

I surrender control.
What I want or don't want is simply an external force trying to cover the hole I feel inside.
I surrender resistance.

The universe is filled with **love** that is flowing to me.
I accept this gift of **love**.

I surrender fear.
The fear of external conditions is a distraction
from this space of pure **love**.

I surrender worry.
Love is so much greater, no matter how
insurmountable it all seems.
This feeling of **love** guides me every step of the way.

I surrender to a higher power,
releasing expectations and the desire to control
specific outcomes.
I allow **love** to flow through me.

With each breath,
surrendering dissolves all fear,
and I allow the expansion of **love** in me.

Create an affirmation card with words you can say to yourself whenever you want to relieve your mind of unnecessary worry and embrace peaceful acceptance. Decide today to let your radiant vibration outshine all "what if" fear.

Laughter Cleanse

Laughing is better than any makeup.
—Unknown

As part of my self-love journey, I created fun and new experiences for rest and rejuvenation. I did anything that made my soul sing, like learning to cook bulgogi (a popular Korean meat dish), riding my bike through Manhattan, and taking a laughing-therapy class led by comedian Thomas Cock. This last one has since become an essential key to living with an elevated vibration.

Laughing is an antiaging elixir that infuses our life with playful energy and instantly boosts your radiant vibration. Studies show that hearty belly laughter can relieve tension and stress, help reduce heart attack and stroke risks, and strengthen the immune system. By laughing more, we boost happy hormones like serotonin and dopamine, which increase our productivity and pleasure. Shared laughter has even been linked to a relationship's well-being and closeness. And let's not forget the beauty of laugh lines; they are a symbol of joy and blissful times.

I was expecting Cock to lead a funny class that made me laugh, but it turned out to be a profound lesson in letting go of what weighs us down. He shared that children laugh between two hundred and three hundred times per day, while adults laugh only twenty to thirty times. As we grow up, we allow stress, worry, and frustrations to weigh us down; we lose our playful spirit along the way. Laughter can be a powerful healing tonic for wounds, pain, and stress. The seriousness dissipates; you let go of "what is," become lighter, and elevate your radiant vibration. While laughter is best experienced spontaneously, this next ritual will help you to carve out time and prioritize fun in your life.

RITUAL: Laughter Cleanse

To feel lighter

Time: 5–10 minutes
Ingredients: Comfortable and safe environment
Optional Upgrades: Journal and pen
Notes: Once you've tried this laughter cleanse, make sure to schedule in time to laugh regularly, especially when you want to raise your radiant vibration.

1. List. Create a list of activities that make you laugh: watching funny movies and stand-up comedy shows, exchanging funny stories with friends, taking a laughing class, listening to a witty podcast, watching YouTube videos of humorous moments.

2. Plan. Carve out time during the week to commit to a "laughter cleanse" activity.

3. Laugh. Even if you don't feel like it, breathe out with laughter and let it go. Cock says that at first, the laughter may feel forced, but it's okay— pretty soon you will begin laughing naturally. If you can laugh until you cry, there's nothing more exhilarating than a laugh and tear cleanse!

4. Affirm. Create an affirmation, such as, *"I laugh and feel light!"* You can add this to your affirmations deck.

Your Radiant Vibration Plan

1. Customize. Decide which rituals you will do this week. My suggestion is to try them all and then choose those that resonate. Commit to doing them at least three times this week.

   - VIBRATIONAL DEEP CLEANSE (to detox stressors and reactions)
   - SELF-LOVE ROLL + GLOW (to release emotional tension)
   - "I SURRENDER" MEDITATION (to let go of "what if" fears)
   - LAUGHTER CLEANSE (to feel lighter)

2. Record. On your phone, record some of the meditations that you've enjoyed, so that you can listen and feel transported whenever you do the rituals.

3. **Schedule.** Write in your planner or put in a GCcal reminder when you will do these rituals. Remember that scheduling in rituals prioritizes *you*!

4. **Cleanse.** And don't forget, wash your face at night while saying your affirmations!

5. **Affirm.** Create three to five self-worth affirmations. Write them on sticky notes, in your journal, or add to your affirmations deck.

6. **Love.** Schedule a self-love activity that elevates your radiant vibration.

CLARIFY YOUR VISION

I recommend doing the rituals in this chapter in consecutive order. Unlike the previous chapters, this one is a cumulative journey. There are three rituals this week, and I've labeled them Parts I, II, and III for clarity. You may experience resistance because this is where the rubber hits the road. But I promise, if you stick with it, you will see the magic unfold. Most importantly, have fun and savor the process!

first became aware of the term "manifesting" during my maid of honor's speech at my wedding in Burgundy, France, when she said, "Angela has the gift of manifesting whatever she wants. She wanted a candlelit wedding in a French château, complete with a horse and carriage. And here we all are, enjoying it!" I got goose bumps as she hugged me. She raised her glass to the guests, who included my kindergarten teacher, Brooklyn landlord and his wife, and college friends, who all smiled and nodded their heads in agreement, as if to say, "Yes, she sure knows how to make things happen."

Long before I understood the nuances of this magical manifesting practice, it seemed to the outside world that I instinctively knew how to turn water into wine, no matter how forced or manufactured my emotional state secretly was at the time. After all, manifesting is a skill that has allowed me to launch multiple businesses, live in my dream city, and create financial stability. But I've also learned that manifesting *things* is not what brings happiness and fulfillment. In the past, I'd disregarded my emotional, physical, and spiritual well-being in the name of attaining "success." As a result, bringing goals to fruition didn't feel as fulfilling as it should have, because I was focused solely on the outcome versus nourishing my radiant feelings during the process.

Over the years, my relationship with manifesting has evolved. It began with → *Bring dreams into reality,* and then shifted to → *Create a life you love*, and now → *Radiate a desired feeling.* Please read that again, because the differences are subtle yet enormously significant.

Manifestations are always an overflow of how you feel during the process of asking the universe for what you desire. For example, at Savor Beauty, we could simply make a goal of creating great skincare products to sell to thousands of customers. But instead, we radiate a desired *feeling* of love and passion, which leads to a business bubbling over with those very sentiments. We employ women who believe in our self-care mission and ethos. They infuse every aspect of their work with care—from making the skincare, to shipping it worldwide. Our customers have expressed how much they not only love the products, but the depth of our mission. What they are responding to isn't just the bona fide business that we've built, but the charisma, light, and radiance that come along with vibrating what we desire.

As I mentioned earlier, I used to think that the purpose of manifesting was to "bring dreams into reality." But while this is an exciting goal, it does not focus on how our souls are aligned with our happiness or how we will ultimately feel when our dreams materialize. It also doesn't relate to how much we will enjoy the actual process of manifesting our future. So, yes, I manifested my dream wedding in the French countryside, but I felt incredibly stressed and strained while planning it. I was able to bring about my vision, but I discounted how important it was to find meaning and fulfillment in the process—which made the wedding less enjoyable for me.

"Create a life you love" is a more holistic manifesting statement and goal than "bring dreams into reality," because it indicates that we love what we manifest. Had I focused on "create a life you love," while planning my wedding, perhaps I would have savored the ceremony, reception, and guests without constantly being worried about details or timing. Even so, "create a life you love" still focuses on the end result, as if that is all that matters to a rich and satisfying life.

I now resonate most with the intention to "radiate a desired feeling," because it puts the focus on sending out an emotion that carries a certain vibration. From here,

I believe that this feeling will not only help others, but bring about a desire that elicits the emotion I want to experience. When you emit and exude vibrancy from a soul that's aligned with how you want to feel, the universe will match it with opportunities and people with the same frequency. The word "desire" also reflects a firm intention, excitement, and craving for our wish, or want. "Radiate a desired feeling" during the wedding process would have extinguished stress with the aura of love felt by everyone. I would have still had a beautiful wedding, but also savored it much more.

If we vibrate and radiate a desired feeling versus remain attached to a specific outcome, the possibilities are endless. For example, the feelings that I focus on daily are peace, abundance, and beauty—and I try to receive and beam these feelings outward. Perhaps I shouldn't be too surprised, then, that while my partner and I recently vacationed in Miami, I experienced the most majestic sunrises and sunsets that filled me with extraordinary splendor and pleasure. We ate oranges so succulent that the juice dripped down our chins. We soaked in the sun (with a sunhat and SPF!), allowing the rays to penetrate the smile I couldn't erase from my face. This feeling of unlimited happiness came to me in the most unexpected of ways, because I've never been drawn to Florida due to preconceived notions, yet this Sunshine State gave me a joyful gift. Setting aside specific outcomes and instead manifesting our desired feelings can bring riches beyond our wildest imagination from the most unexpected of places.

Manifest What You Radiate

If you want to find the secrets of the universe, think in terms of energy, frequency and vibration.
—**Nikola Tesla, Serbian American inventor and engineer**

A few years after launching my companies, I found myself caught in a whirlwind of having manifested more "outcomes" than I could handle. I wanted to be a supermom, wonder wife, and entrepreneur extraordinaire. Yet I was drowning and felt overwhelmed in the process. I began to feel pulled in all directions. I worked nonstop and fell into the "disease to please" trap. After hosting a major conference in New York City for five hundred women sponsored by American Express, Whole Foods, and Goldman Sachs, it looked from the outside as though I was on top of the world. It seemed so glamorous and successful, but something felt very wrong inside of me. One hot afternoon, as the subway became more crowded with people, I had a frightening panic attack. I could feel my throat closing up, and I gasped, "I am going to throw up! Please give me space!"

My soul was crying out for help, but I did not know how to give it to myself, so after the incident, I kept working harder and attracting more overwhelming situations. And while there were moments of incredible happiness, the responsibilities felt crushing; my body and mental health collapsed. I began to experience the same physical symptoms of burnout that I had when I was a pianist (eczema, itching, burning, intestinal pain, and discomfort), plus panic attacks and insomnia every night.

One of my best friends, Julie, was in a similar situation to mine. I shared a part of her story in week 4, where she encouraged me from her hospital bed to go to Cancun when I felt guilty because I didn't feel that I deserved it. She was running two businesses at the time—a family grocery store and a fashion agency. After the 2020 COVID-19 lockdown in New York City, she was forced to put in double time at the grocery store as an essential business owner. Julie was in work overload, and every time we connected, she was bone-tired.

While she was in the hospital, Julie underwent emergency brain surgery due to a ruptured aneurysm and ended up receiving multiple procedures to try to fix the problem. To make matters worse, Julie had a stroke on top of all this. Work and stress had run Julie into the ground. There were worrisome nights when we did not know if she would make it. When I visited her, I gave her one of my favorite amethyst crystals to hold, and read chapters to her from *The Magic* by Rhonda Byrne.

Miraculously, Julie made a turn for the better and was released from the hospital two months later. I was so grateful to have my best friend back, and to help her rebuild, I asked her to do a visioning session with me, which is something we always did together. I noticed, though, that she'd become uncharacteristically quiet, and days later when I checked in to see how she was doing, she texted, "I'm sorry. I just can't do any visioning now. I'm all over the place. Sometimes I'm happy. Other times, my head and emotions go to a dark place. I feel I can't manifest anything until I feel joy again."

When I visited Julie shortly after, we talked about radiating a positive, desired feeling to attract like frequencies. I shared my story about being broke in my twenties and walking around saying, "I'm rich in all ways" until I could feel the energy of these words in my bones. It helped me over the years to turn things around and attract amazing grace in love, friendship, and finances. Julie's eyes brightened, and she told me she wanted to vibrate and radiate ease and joy. This is precisely where she needed to start, and even though it seemed basic, it was a powerful reminder that manifesting always begins with nourishing our radiance, vibration, and energy.

Today, I'm happy to report that Julie is well and meditates daily to find her center, which I believe to be the major reason she is in good health. Let our stories be of inspiration to you. Working and succeeding with the wrong intention will magnetize stress and illness. Tune in to your radiance, allow it to swirl in and around you, and let this be the positive intention that is your guiding force for every manifestation that you aim to create.

RITUAL (Part I): Radiance Meditation

To meditate on and radiate your desired feeling

Time: 30 minutes

Ingredients: Pen, paper, recording device (I use my iPhone), face cleanser, and moisturizer

Optional Upgrades: Background music, fresh flowers, candles, crystals

Notes: Remember that you are not writing about a specific outcome. You are describing a feeling vibration that you wish to radiate, a reflection of your beauty, intuition, and best self.

1. **Cleanse.** Thoroughly wash your face with a gentle cleanser, taking care to cleanse every pore. Pat and dry your face with a clean towel, and hydrate your skin with your favorite moisturizer for a glowing complexion.

2. **Breathe.** Take a seat in a space where you can think and write comfortably. Take a loving inhale,

filling your belly with fresh air. Exhale. Repeat until you feel relaxed and focused.

3. Write. Use the following script as a guide to write your own meditation, which you will record onto your phone. I've provided prompts and used the word "love" as the intended vibration; feel free to replace this with your own intended vibration and personalize the italicized words.

[your name],
Let's breathe in and out three times, counting to four.
Inhale, 2, 3, 4.
Hold, 2, 3, 4.
Exhale, 2, 3, 4.
[Repeat 2 more times.]

Imagine a beautifully soft, warm, radiant, and loving energy surrounding you.
It feels healing as you bask in this white healing aura and vibration.
Your ability to manifest is powerful.

You have *love* flowing in and to you.
Love feels . . .
happy
joyful

flowing
freeing
abundant.

Every action you take is in alignment with
happiness
joy
flow
freedom
ease.

You are bathing in this vibration of *love*.
You're playful and lighthearted about life.
You feel good, unconditionally.
This vibration of *love* is flowing from your radiant
source and filling you up.
You are radiating *love* from inside out.
It's a magnetic energy that's so warm.
It magnetizes like frequency, and you are manifesting
with *love*,
Strong and soft
Feminine and powerful.
It's loving, delicious, and you are manifesting with
this intended vibration.

It's a feeling of *abundance, joy, peace.*
This vibration of *love* feels *nourishing, gorgeous, light,*

playful,
And, [your name], it is yours.

4. **Record.** Record yourself reading the meditation in a soft, hypnotic voice. You can play your favorite music or nature sounds in the background to create a soothing spalike environment.
5. **Listen.** Access this meditation whenever you want to radiate your intended vibration.
6. **Appreciate.** Feel gratitude for what is and what's to come. Write or state it out loud.
7. **Affirm.** Create an affirmation to add to your affirmation deck, journal, or a sticky note. Make sure it's easily accessible so you can read it daily or as needed. You can extract your favorite phrase from the meditation and turn it into an affirmation. For example:

"I have love flowing in and around me."

Manifest Wheel

Creativity is the state of consciousness in which you enter into the treasury of your innermost being and bring the beauty into manifestation.

—Torkom Saraydarian, Armenian American musician and spiritual teacher

Five years ago, my Instagram bio read, "Mom, wife, founder." This was my identity in three punchy, concise words, and my days were spent mom-ing, wife-ing, and boss-ing. I had zero concept of what life balance meant, and to be honest, whenever people talked about the need to feel more balanced, I secretly harbored cynical thoughts that balance was a myth. I rarely invested in developing, much less viewing, myself as a whole person, and this led to severe burnout as a mom, wife, and boss. I constantly gave from an empty cup to everyone but myself.

Years later, when I began my quest for self-love, I swung in the far opposite direction by vacationing, relaxing, and nourishing my soul as much as I could. The coronavirus pandemic also forced me to spend time with fewer people. In many ways, it was refreshing and rejuvenating, but I also realized that I received great satisfaction from my work and in connecting with others as well. To discover and honor all aspects of my being, I created a Manifest Wheel with six different areas in life: self-care, soul-care, success, social, space, and savoring life.

Each category on my wheel had an equal-sized slice that collectively added up to a balanced and whole life. While investing the same amount of time in each category isn't always realistic, the more we give them equal thought and reinforce the feelings behind them, the more purposefully we bring to life the different expressions of ourselves. Creating a Manifest Wheel and practicing being whole helps

Manifest Wheel
Beauty, Brilliance, Balance

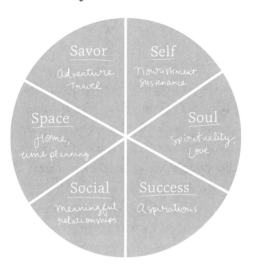

you radiate balance and revel in the richness of your *entire* being.

Here is a breakdown of what each category meant to me, and soon, will mean to you, too:

1. **Self-care:** This category includes self-discovery and all that helps us to thrive: beauty rituals, body health, mental health, food choices, exercise, and personal style.
2. **Soul-care:** What feeds your soul and makes it

sing? Here, think spirituality, meditation, creativity, love, and passion.

3. **Success:** Feeling successful brings forth confidence in the arenas of career, finances, education, skills, or other aspirations.

4. **Social:** Studies show that deep and meaningful relationships are the key to happiness. Connections and support can come from friends, family, community, and charitable work.

5. **Space:** This category includes creating an aesthetically pleasing, healthy, organized, safe, and supportive home environment.

6. **Savor life:** Vacations, adventures, and fun! This category restores balance in life with unplugged time to replenish your radiance.

RITUAL (Part II): Create Your Manifest Wheel

To clarify your desires

Time: 60 minutes

Ingredients: Pen, paper, vision board or journal, a facial toning mist of choice

Optional Upgrades: Background music, candle, essential oils

Notes: Light a candle, turn on your favorite music, and enjoy the process of allowing your right brain to take over for this activity. Beyond creating your Manifest Wheel, this exercise's real power is in creating balance to radiate through your whole being.

1. **Balance.** Mist your face three times with a balancing toner, such as neroli, which is known to help maintain the right moisture and oil balance in the skin (my favorite is Savor Beauty's Neroli Toning Mist). It also has a sensual orange-blossom scent that helps restore balance and an inner sense of calm.

2. **Reflect.** Create your own Manifest Wheel, and do a brain dump of what comes to mind for each pie slice in the circle. I've included thought-starters to get your juices flowing:

   a. **Self-care:** How can you take better care of yourself? What brings out your best self?

   b. **Soul-care:** What feeds your soul and makes it sing? How can you connect to your soul? This can include meditation, creativity, and spirituality.

   c. **Success:** How do you want to flourish in career or finances? What are your personal or professional aspirations? Do you want to develop new skills or take a course?

   d. **Social:** Is there anyone with whom you want to spend more time—from loved ones to acquaintances? How do you want to expand your network? Sometimes we forget nourishing people that we meet in our daily lives. Spend more time with them!

 e. **Space:** Is your space pleasing to you? What would make your home, in the words of Oprah Winfrey, "rise up to greet you"? What would make it nourishing, calming, soothing, and a place of replenishment and restoration?

 f. **Savor life:** Is there a dream vacation that you have been wanting to plan? Any adventures, excursions you want to take, or fun activities you want to do?

3. **Appreciate.** Now, what are you grateful for as you look at your Manifest Wheel? State what you appreciate as you develop and integrate all aspects of your evolving self.

4. **Affirm.** Create an affirmation that reminds you to honor your whole self. Add it to your affirmation deck, journal, or a sticky note so you can access it as needed. For example:

"I honor and appreciate the full beauty of who I am."
"I express and live out all aspects of myself."

Next, we'll create Radiance Intentions to build on your Manifest Wheel.

Radiance Intentions

Create the highest, grandest vision possible for your life, because you become what you believe.
—Oprah Winfrey

Now we will take your Manifest Wheel and use it as a base to create Radiance Intentions, which are guiding principles and statements of purpose that you want to align yourself with, rather than a fixed goal. They come from the heart and are driven by a desire to connect with our authentic selves. I purposefully create Radiance Intentions that don't necessarily lock in a tangible outcome, because I like to leave room for miracles and spontaneous surprises. As I always say to my daughter, "Aim for the stars, but there's always the moon, too."

A business always has a mission statement, and I've come to believe that our lives should have an empowering vision statement, too. We are visionaries of our lives, so it makes sense that this statement is a representation of the values and philosophies that we choose to integrate and express in our lives. A good Radiance Intention reverberates high-vibration feelings and first lives in our minds, then on our lips, and, soon enough, in the external world as a manifestation.

I like for a Radiance Intention to sound like it's a delicious dessert that you crave—appealing to every one of your senses. We want to feel drawn to read these words every day and to feel, see, touch, smell, and taste them. Allow these manifestos to inspire, resonate, and revive us. They are celebrations of us as *whole* beings in a world of our own creation.

Here are some examples of my Radiance Intentions to inspire your own. You'll notice that the categories listed here are the same as those on the Manifest Wheel. The more you reinforce and expand on your goals and the feelings behind them, the more likely it is that they'll manifest.

Self-Care

My motto is "Easy, breezy." I nourish my radiance and attract the high-vibration frequencies. I make mindful choices about my health, well-being, and happiness. I embrace my feminine energy, and my body feels free. My soul is an oasis of peace and beauty, which radiates as a healing source for those around me.

Soul-Care

My daughter is thriving as a happy being. She is engaged in her passions and tries her best in school. I am a calm and loving presence, which helps her to discover and be who she is. She feels heard and loved. She feels cared for and guided. She has healthy self-esteem and is kind, grateful, and loving. She's my best friend, and I'm so proud of that girl!!!

I'm in a connected, passionate, committed relationship with my best friend and lover. We have magical chemistry, connection, and compatibility. We are each other's rocks and have an unshakable foundation of joie de vivre, trust, honesty, openness, warmth, lovemaking, generosity, support, respect, appreciation, life adventure. It feels so easy and effortless to go deep and wide in this ocean of love.

Success

I'm writing a book about self-love with ease and inspiration, as messages flow through me. The book brings hope and healing to those who are searching to infuse their lives with self-love radiance. I'm the vessel that allows messages to come through my heart, soul, and wisdom.

Savor Beauty is a brand that provides nourishing high-vibration products and rituals to millions of people worldwide. I feel honored and humbled to help our customers radiate their authentic beauty.

Social

I have an abundance of friends I love and adore. I am here for them; they are here for me—lots of meals with stimulating conversations, toasting champagne for life celebrations, connected support for one another. My man and I meet new and old friends and stay in touch. It feels like discovering rare jewels and appreciating them for life!

Space

I have a gorgeous modern apartment with luxurious
space, healing spalike environment, inspiring views,
gorgeous sunlight, stylish decor, cozy rooms,
outdoor space with greenery and summer lights.
I make time in this sacred space for sweet love,
friends, family, laughter, memories, meditation, cooking,
cozy teas, morning coffee, music, writing, dancing, and
more!

Savor Life

I'm traveling around the world with loved ones, savoring
delicious local food, making new friends, experiencing
local culture, basking in the sun (with sun hat and SPF!) on
a beach discovering new wonders. I bring back renewing
rituals to infuse into life, allowing each travel journey
to reset and rejuvenate mind, body, and spirit for years to
come.

You will notice that my Radiance Intentions are not focused on fixed goals. I want to open myself to the miracles
of what these feeling intentions will magnetize, so I focus
on emotions and values.

The rules for creating Radiance Intentions are similar to affirmations, so I will highlight what we covered
before:

1. Phrase Radiance Intentions in the present tense.
2. State your intentions in the positive.
3. Attach a feeling to your intention.

Now it's time to create your own Radiance Intentions! After doing the following ritual, be sure to carve out time to read, speak, listen, study, love, and savor these words. Soon, they will be part of who you are.

RITUAL (Part III): Create Your Radiance Intentions

To attract what you desire

Time: 60 minutes

Ingredients: Pen and paper or sticky notes, or a digital device, your Manifest Wheel

Optional Upgrades: Candle, crystals, inspiring music

Notes: Print your Manifest Wheel so that you can easily reference it. Your Radiance Intentions are works in progress, so don't worry about making them perfect! You will reflect and refine them over time. Make your intentions easily accessible so you can meditate on these visions daily.

1. **Brain dump.** Begin writing out Radiance Intentions for each section of your Manifest Wheel. What do you desire? How would it make you feel? Feel free to include the following:
   a. Inspiring motto or quotes
   b. High-vibration words
   c. Emotions and feelings
   d. Things that spark the imagination
   e. Playful emojis
   f. Gratitude and appreciation

2. **Meditate.** Carve out time to meditate on these intentional statements daily.

3. **Listen.** Record your intentions and listen to them daily during meditation, while exercising, or before falling asleep.

4. **Edit.** As you read your intentions, feel free to tweak, change, and elevate them!

5. **Affirm.** Create a message from your Higher Self to affirm these statements, such as, *"I love saying my Radiance Intentions daily."* Add it to your affirmations deck.

6. **Appreciate.** Fall in love with these Radiance Intentions. They are a reflection of your beauty, intuition, and best self. Feel gratitude for what is and what's to come.

7. **Feel.** As I've said so many times throughout this

book, when you read or listen to your intentions, *feel* the vibrancy of each word. This will help you magnetize with ease and power.

Radiance Intentions are such powerful tools for manifesting, so I suggest creating a system to remember doing them. My partner has an adorable little method to remember his daily rituals: he created the acronym GIMP, which stands for gratitude, intentions, meditation, and push-ups.

Your Vision Plan

1. **Schedule.** I recommend doing the rituals in consecutive order. Unlike most other chapters, this one is a cumulative journey.
   - I. RADIANCE MEDITATION (to radiate what you want to attract)
   - II. CREATE YOUR MANIFEST WHEEL (to clarify your desires)
   - III. CREATE YOUR RADIANCE INTENTIONS (to create a clear written statement)
2. **Plan.** Write in your planner or put in a GCal reminder when you will do these rituals. Remember that scheduling in rituals prioritizes *you*!
3. **Cleanse.** Don't forget to cleanse and hydrate your skin at night while saying your affirmations!

4. **Affirm.** Create three to five self-worth affirmations. Write them on sticky notes, in your journal, or add to your affirmations deck. Something like, *"I own my worth. I see my worth. I am worth it."*

5. **Love.** Schedule a self-love activity that elevates your radiant vision.

GROW LITTLE BY LITTLE

I recommend doing the "Grow Little by Little" rituals in consecutive order, as you did in chapter 7, as this is also a cumulative journey.

I n the last chapter, we mapped out our Manifest Wheel and Radiance Intentions. Keeping the feelings and desires in mind that you set out to manifest in the last chapter, we're now going to create an activation plan using various tools, including a ninety-day plan, weekly plan, and daily rituals. These fun and simple exercises will help you specify and outline the baby steps that support your manifestation efforts. The process of manifestation is as much about setting the right intention as it is about taking baby action steps. I find it thrilling to tune in to my radiant source and then step into the action mode. Both feed into each other and bring a sense of euphoria and joy that one gets from turning nothing into something.

I will never forget the remarkable manifestation lesson that I learned from a dear college friend named Paul Merkelo, who is the principal trumpet player of the Montreal

Symphony Orchestra, one of the top ten orchestras in the world. While preparing to perform one of the hardest solos in Symphony no. 5 by Gustav Mahler, Paul initially confided that he felt a tremendous amount of pressure to deliver a "perfect" performance (as a perfectionist myself, I could relate).

Even so, Paul pulled it off masterfully—and when I marveled at his skill and composure, he let me in on the secret to his admirable success. "Learning something as big as the Mahler symphony is like conquering a huge boulder," he said. "If I look at the entire boulder, I stop dead in my tracks. So with the big vision in mind, I put on my blinders and chip away at it, every day, a little bit at a time. Then at the performance, I don't even realize I've conquered that big boulder. It's just a thousand tiny chips that I've polished, and it's part of my blood and bones. At the time of the performance, the piece is not what I have to do. It's *who I am*."

When Paul shared his MO, I was so inspired that I began applying it to my own goals. Paul didn't allow himself to drown in the big picture of an overwhelming symphony. He broke down his vision and accomplished all of its important details, little by little, which is a technique we can all apply to whatever we set out to accomplish, too. If you chip away at a large task, every day, much like Paul did, your efforts won't feel laborious; they will become part of you.

Hold the Space

"Love" is the name for our pursuit of wholeness,
for our desire to be complete.

—Plato

Before we create your ninety-day, weekly, and daily rituals, I want to share a concept with you called "hold the space." Holding the space means to carve out time to focus on our visions, prime the environment, get rid of distractions, and accomplish tasks. It's the intention to carve out space in our minds—and schedules—to manifest our desires. I like to hold the space in seven-minute increments because often the hardest part is getting started on any project. If I tell myself, "It's only for seven minutes," I'm more likely to commit than if I feel like I have hours of work ahead of me.

It's challenging to get started on anything if you don't feel inspired or motivated, especially if you're already faced with other mundane tasks on your to-do list. You may not feel like meditating to get into your zen. Or feel called to exercise. Or inspired to spend the next six hours at your computer. As if that weren't inhibiting enough, if you approach your work with uninspired vibrations, they have the potential to manifest into the very opposite of what you desire. For example, let's say that you have a job interview you are nervous about, and you want to begin preparing. Using the energy of dread and criticism to prepare, versus that of curiosity and openness, could produce less-than-optimal results because of the low vibrations these feelings carry. Fueling your efforts with high-vibing energy will always open more doors to your desires.

My favorite example of what it means to hold space happens in yoga class. While sitting calmly on your mat, have you ever thought, "This feels amazing! But I have a yoga mat at home. Why don't I do this on my own?" The reason is that your yoga instructor has held the space for you through affirmations and guidance, making the session enjoyable. She's planned your routine, carved out time, and primed the environment by having the best yoga tools ready. There are no distractions, and you intend to be fully present. By the end of the class, you feel rejuvenated and restored. Holding space has made your efforts feel effortless.

Sometimes we feel inspired to act, and sometimes our actions inspire us. Spiritually speaking, we need to do for ourselves what the yoga instructor does for her students. Holding space in the right environment—with the proper tools and no distractions—invites an easy, creative, intuitive, and focused energy to flow through you that helps you get started without feeling overwhelmed. And if you think about holding the space for a short time at first, say seven minutes, it makes it easier to begin the larger undertaking. Sometimes during those seven minutes, I feel like stopping, but think, "I only have three minutes left. I can do this!" Then I take a break—make a smoothie, do some stretches, talk to a friend, water the plants—before I start up again. Sometimes I get a little bit done, which makes me feel better than doing nothing and feeling stagnant. But most of the time, I build momentum during those key seven minutes, and before I know it, an hour of inspired momentum has passed. It's all about growing, little by little, and I promise—the result is life-changing!

RITUAL: Hold the Space

To nourish and nurture your desires

Time: 7 minutes

Ingredients: Timer, all tools needed to accomplish your desired goal, undistracted environment

Notes: This little seven-minute secret will get you started on any activity, from washing dishes, to exercising, to working on a big project. It will help you achieve them in doable bursts of time and energy. There are other techniques, such as the Pomodoro Technique, that encourage twenty-five-minute increments, but for me, seven minutes is the perfect amount of time to motivate me to begin. You can also start by doing an activity, three minutes at a time, and work your way up to seven. When the timer rings, you have the choice to stop or continue. You'll be surprised at the momentum you build!

1. **Prime.** Make sure your environment is free of all distractions, to set yourself up for success. Go to a private space, gather your tools, and put away technical devices you aren't using.

2. **Breathe.** Inhale one deep breath in while saying to yourself, *"Open."* Exhale slowly while reciting an affirmative word. I say, *"Possibility"* or *"Focus."*

3. **Intend.** State in one simple sentence what you want to hold the space for. For example:

    "I intend to enjoy creating designs at work."
    "I hold the space to journal for seven minutes."

4. **Hold.** Set your timer for seven minutes and allow yourself to become immersed in the work for seven glorious minutes.

5. **Ask.** At the end of the seven minutes, ask yourself how you feel and then decide if you will continue with another seven minutes. If you feel inspired momentum, you can stop the timer and stay in the zone for as long as you desire.

6. **Affirm.** At the end of your session, affirm your creativity and dedication:

    "Being creative and productive feels amazing!"

The Quarterly Ritual: Ninety-Day Vision

Ninety days from now, you will thank yourself for having started.

—Sara Blette, designer

One of my time-tested ways of holding space is to create a ninety-day vision based on how I want to feel and what desires I want to manifest. I used to create ten-year plans and annual goals, but I've learned that when you make plans, the universe laughs. For example, if you would have told me a decade ago that I would retire from my piano career and launch a beauty business, I would have thought you were joking. It's so important to stay flexible and open to the surprises that life has in store for you.

So today I prefer to plan my life in what I call ninety-day "bursts of joy." I revisit my Manifest Wheel and Radiance Intentions (from chapter 7), subsequently planning for only the next three months. Starting a new vision every quarter is like having four New Year's resolutions in a year, with plenty of time to hold the space to reflect, stay the course, and refine my aspirations. Ninety days is also a perfectly doable time frame—not too short or too long. You can create enough momentum during this time, but also make small shifts if you want to change course.

I also believe in the power of other people growing little by little with you: I call them accountability partners. From 2014 to 2019, I ran a ninety-day vision program called Savor Success Circles, which thousands of women participated in. The intention was to help them create their ninety-day visions and match them to three like-minded women with similar goals to support one another for three months. For instance, four women launching businesses met virtually once a week to help each other with each phase of their launches. It was beautiful to see thousands of women enjoy supporting each other and developing lifelong friendships. In fact, I still get emails from them sharing their stories of how their "Savor Sisters" have become best friends while helping each other through major milestones.

In the same vein, while you can create your ninety-day vision on your own, I encourage you to have fun refining your goals with like-minded souls. You can even host a ninety-day vision party with up to six guests (or just yourself!), in person or virtually. It's easy and fun, especially when you turn on your favorite music, light candles, and follow the ritual directions listed.

RITUAL: Create Your Ninety-Day Vision

To make a fresh start every ninety days

Time: 30–60 minutes

Ingredients: Pen and paper, a digital device, or the *Savor Beauty Planner*

Notes: In the previous chapter, we created your Manifest Wheel and Radiance Intentions, which you will use in this ritual as references. It's best to complete them in advance of this ritual. If you are doing this ritual solo, you may want to make an afternoon, day, or even weekend of it! You could do this ritual during a spa day or mini getaway for breathing room.

1. **Breathe.** Inhale and exhale mindfully until you feel centered and grounded.
2. **Reflect.** When looking back on your last ninety days, ask yourself:
   a. What have I learned in the last ninety days?
   b. What's been flowing in the last ninety days?
   c. What's not been flowing in the last ninety days?
   d. What do I want to do the same or differently?
3. **Affirm.** What feeling do you want to radiate in the next ninety days? Remember, you radiate and attract

what you feel. Create an affirmation or choose a theme!

4. **Reset.** Look at your Manifest Wheel and Radiance Intentions. Are you in alignment with your desires? Remember that you are always evolving. Honor the evolution and edit accordingly.

5. **Desire.** What do you want to manifest in the next ninety days? What do you want to accomplish during that time? Let go of what no longer feels aligned, and take what's working to make it a focal point for the next ninety days.

6. **Visualize.** Feel free to cut and paste an inspiring visual next to your vision. Commit to meditating on your vision and how you want to feel every day.

The Weekly Ritual: Mind Detox

The journey of a thousand miles begins with a single step.

—**Lao Tzu**

Once your ninety-day vision is complete, you will be able to refer back to it each week to make sure that your actions are in alignment with your intentions so that you can manifest your goals with ease. So let's start taking bites out of your to-do list by beginning with what I call a Mind Detox ritual. I call it a "detox" because you are literally dumping out the "good, bad, and ugly" to-dos—everything from miscellaneous to vision-oriented tasks—from your brain. I love to do Mind Detoxes on Sundays, because it's great to begin the week with renewed intentions and purposeful planning. I enjoy taking a purifying salt bath, shopping for the week's meals, and then diving into my Mind Detox to enter the week feeling refreshed.

A Mind Detox is similar to a skin detox: it purifies, heals, and clarifies. Have you ever thought of things you need to do and then felt guilty when you didn't accomplish them? Nothing drains energy more than your "do this, do that" inner voice. Studies show that getting "to-dos" out of the head and onto paper is therapeutic and cathartic; it feels like an emotional purge. It dampens anxiety, gives you structure, and boosts confidence to know there's a plan in place.

Getting things done has a masculine, pushing energy to it, as we discussed in chapter 5; however, we can use our feminine energy by tapping into our natural flow of inspiration and nourishment. As I've mentioned, these are little actions for which your future self will thank you—the ultimate act of self-love. Shift your mindset to one that views the tasks as beneficial to your well-being rather than as an emotional or mental drain.

For example, let's say I need to make a doctor's appointment for an annual visit. Instead of framing it as a dreaded task, I would approach it as the pathway to greater health and well-being. My future self would thank my past self for having taken the steps necessary to manifest what I ultimately desire.

Every Sunday, I like to go to a café, order a cortado or mimosa during brunch, and take out my planner. Here's an example of what might be in my Mind Detox list for the week:

- Create a wish list of ingredients for a new SPF face lotion.
- Make an Instagram video to show how I wash my face at night.
- Storyboard self-love package to send to beauty editors.
- Sign up for breath-work class.
- Pick up flowers.
- Buy daughter new shoes.
- Decide meals for the week.
- Order groceries.
- Send mom a coffee gift.
- Invite Carolyn to dinner at home.

Sometimes I have to sit for a while to get inspired to set my plans for the week. I flip back to previous Mind Detox lists to see what I've missed, think about upcoming commitments, draw and doodle—anything to get the juices flowing. Once you have your to-dos and tasks on paper, it feels good to know where you're headed. It's like a spiritual cleanse for mind and soul.

RITUAL: Weekly Mind Detox

To start each week feeling calm and poised, or for when you feel overwhelmed

Time: 15–30 minutes

Ingredients: Pen and notebook, a digital organizer, or the *Savor Beauty Planner*

Notes: Give yourself the gift of time and space with this ritual on your weekly day(s) off. Refer back to this living and breathing document every week to stay authentically aligned with your priorities.

1. **Breathe.** Breathe in and out with your eyes closed.
2. **Affirm.** Say a grounding affirmation like, *"This week is filled with possibilities and opportunities coming my way."*
3. **Write.** Begin writing anything that comes to mind that you need to get done. You can divide your sheet of paper into different areas of your life—for example, work, personal, self-care.
4. **Refer.** If you keep your Mind Detox lists in a planner, refer back to your lists and rewrite important tasks that didn't get accomplished.
5. **Prioritize.** Clarify the top three priorities of the week. If you don't get anything else done this

week, at least you can hold the space for your
priorities.

6. **Self-care.** Highlight something that you will
do for yourself this week. Remember: *Nourish to
flourish!*

Pull Weeds

*For each new morning, let there be flow of love. Let
there be light of happiness in every direction.*
—Dr. Amit Ray, Indian author and spiritual master

My dad had an incredible work ethic and taught me to always wake up early to get work done first thing in the morning. This allows you to get your unappealing tasks finished
first, so you can then enjoy the rest of the day. I adopted this
philosophy as a pianist and laid out my practice schedule accordingly. Even though I was tempted to start playing Mozart
and Ravel because I loved those composers, I'd always first
tackle the pieces I didn't like practicing so I could move past
them and on to my favorites. Getting the challenging or less
enjoyable music out of the way at the top of the morning
gave me so much to look forward to, like dessert after a meal!

I like to refer to the process of first doing the stuff that
you like least as "pulling weeds" in your metaphorical garden. Pulling weeds is an important task that needs to get

done, but it's often the most difficult or unpleasant. You wrote a lot of these kinds of tasks down on your Weekly Mind Detox list, and now we are going to break them into daily activities, or weeds. For example, maybe your least favorite weeds are paying bills, scheduling appointments, or doing taxes. These are the nonglamorous activities you often procrastinate over or don't want to handle. And left unattended, your garden will become unruly, messy, and chaotic. But if you pull these weeds on a daily basis, you will actually enjoy the clearing process so that your garden can blossom with beautiful flowers.

I think of weeds as the operational or logistical tasks that are not the most energizing tasks on our lists, but they bring simplicity and ease to life. For example:

- Open mail.
- Organize paperwork.
- Clean out the closet.
- Visit vet for pet's annual shots.
- Do laundry.
- Reconcile financial statements.
- Choose outfits for the week.
- Do homework.
- Paint bedroom.
- Get oil changed.
- Renew passport.
- Deep-clean fridge.

We often want to procrastinate these to-dos, but the sooner you get them done, the sooner you can savor and enjoy your day.

RITUAL: Pull Weeds Daily
To start every day feeling calm and organized

Time: Up to 1 hour, daily

Ingredients: Pen and paper, a digital device, or the *Savor Beauty Planner*

Notes: It's best to pull a few weeds daily to keep overwhelm at bay. Try to hold the space for weed pulling in the morning so that you can enjoy the rest of the day! I refer to my Weekly Mind Detox list to make sure I don't miss anything. Then I create a week's view from Monday to Friday and list three weeds a day that need to go.

1. **Write.** Start by writing down three weeds that you need to pull daily. Refer to your Weekly Mind Detox list, or ask yourself, "What are some tasks I've been procrastinating about?"

2. **Affirm.** Create an intention before you start, such as, *"I create ease in my life."*

3. **Pull.** If it's challenging to get started on pulling your weeds, set a seven-minute timer and hold the space for momentum.

4. **Check.** Have a check-mark party! Studies show that checking things off your list gives you a sense of accomplishment and the motivation to keep going.

Plant Seeds

I love the smell of possibility in the morning.
—Unknown

The opposite of pulling weeds is "planting seeds." For me, planting seeds is a daily ritual that is on par with washing my face: both have the most profound impact for nourishing radiance. Planting seeds is any action that has the potential for personal or professional growth, such as connecting with colleagues, applying for a new opportunity, or taking a new class. If there is one ritual that brings and replenishes abundance, it's planting seeds. When I first started creating lotions and potions in my kitchen, I planted multiple seeds every day. I called different farmers and asked questions about their ingredients. I purchased various ingredients, such as rose hip, evening primrose, and pumpkin, to test which ones felt the best on the skin. I went to Whole Foods and conducted unofficial tests on random customers to get their blind feedback on which lotions or sugar scrubs they preferred—either my own concoctions or "competitor" brands.

Eventually, I planted hundreds of seeds to start my skincare business. Some didn't grow, while others blossomed. Some seeds took a few minutes to sprout, while others took years. After planting my seeds, I try to detach from the outcome and trust that each flower will bloom when the time is right. Working toward goals and simultaneously letting them go is not giving up; it's creating the freedom and room to allow small and big miracles to flow into our lives.

Planting seeds is an antidote to the fear of rejection and a tonic for confidence. If you don't plant seeds consciously or intentionally, it's easy to become attached to and insecure about random outcomes. If you plant seeds as a daily ritual, you don't become attached to any one outcome and do gain tremendous confidence as you experience a multitude of blossoming seeds.

Prepandemic, all of my seeds were professional. They included pitching a new segment to the QVC producers, traveling to Seoul with my mom and daughter, and planning self-love events with like-minded partnerships. My daily seed list looked like this:

- Schedule walk-and-talk meetings with new staff members.
- Pitch to three beauty editors.
- Connect with QVC buyers.
- Email Seoul contacts.
- Send beauty-event presale accouncement to partners.

When COVID-19 and the New York City lockdown wiped out all of those plans, QVC suspended all of its live segments. I didn't see my mom for over a year. All work and personal events were canceled. So instead of planting seeds to achieve company goals, I began planting seeds that helped me to grow personally. My daily seed list looked more like this:

- Do meditations and *"I am radiant"* affirmations.
- Sign up for virtual Kundalini yoga class.
- Go on socially distanced hikes.
- Read *The Magic* by Rhonda Byrne.

Personal growth translated to business growth, as intuition and balance guided me to make decisions with wisdom and clarity.

RITUAL: Plant Seeds Daily

To grow beautiful abundance and fulfillment

Time: Anywhere from 5 to 60 minutes a day, depending on how much free time you have for this activity

Ingredients: Pen and paper, a digital organizer, or the *Savor Beauty Planner*

Notes: Hold the space to plant seeds in the morning when you feel fresh! As with pulling weeds, I like to create a week's view from Monday to Friday and then list three seeds a day.

1. **Write.** Start by writing down three seeds to plant daily. Refer to your Weekly Mind Detox list for guidance.
2. **Affirm.** Create an intention before you start, such as, *"I plant seeds daily to enjoy an abundant garden."*
3. **Plant.** If it's challenging to get started, set a seven-minute timer and hold the space for momentum.
4. **Appreciate.** Draw a star next to the seeds that blossom, so you can appreciate the abundance!
5. **Nurture.** When you plant a seed, sometimes it

needs daily nourishment. For example, if you sign up for a French class, a daily review of vocabulary words will help your love for, and retention of, the language grow.

Your Growth Plan

1. **Customize.** My suggestion is to try the Hold the Space and Create Your Ninety-Day Vision rituals first. Then proceed with the Weekly Mind Detox, Pull Weeds Daily, and Plant Seeds Daily rituals for the full ninety days.

   - HOLD THE SPACE (to nourish and nurture your desires)
   - CREATE YOUR NINETY-DAY VISION (to get a fresh start every ninety days)
   - WEEKLY MIND DETOX (to start the week feeling calm)
   - PULL WEEDS DAILY (to start the day feeling calm)
   - PLANT SEEDS DAILY (to grow beautiful abundance and fulfillment)

2. **Plan.** Write in your planner or put in a GCal reminder when you will do these rituals. Remember that scheduling in rituals prioritizes *you*!

3. **Cleanse.** Don't forget to cleanse and hydrate your skin at night while saying your affirmations.

4. **Affirm.** Create three to five self-worth affirmations. Write them on sticky notes or in your journal.

5. **Love.** Schedule a self-love activity that elevates your growth.

FLOW WITH MOMENTUM

Manifesting is an important cornerstone of self-love and self-care, because when we do it, we see proof of our innermost desires materializing in the outside world. And as we bring our soul's beautiful cravings to life, what we are really doing is cultivating radiance. It's a radiance that runs deep within us. Now we want to *wear* this radiance and give this light a rhythmic flow that builds and builds, feeding an intensifying momentum. Momentum is declaring an intention and moving in the direction of it. The process is like riding a bike: the left foot achieves "focused desire" and the right foot, "inspired action." If you think back to what we covered in week 2, we defined passion as focused desire. When paired with inspired action, both work in tandem, creating a euphoria, vitalization, and flush of excitement that electrifies our energy field to attract more like frequencies at astounding speed. The combination of these two creates momentum. I have been blown away at how quickly my intentions have manifested when momentum carries me. And the beauty of momentum is that it carries us through good and challenging times, too.

Shortly after people began to get their COVID-19 vaccinations in the spring of 2021, I went to Savor Spa to connect with my manager and suggested that we keep the spa door open to allow the breeze to circulate. Within one hour, at least ten passersby stuck their heads in to welcome us back, purchase products, or book a facial. It was deeply thrilling to feel our customers' happy warmth once again, and it was validation that momentum has lasting effects. Throughout lockdown, we paired focused passion on the business with inspired action by keeping in touch with our customers and providing them with self-care tools through one of the most uncertain periods in my company's history. To use the analogy of riding a bike, as we revved up to reopen our spas, the momentum of focused desire and inspired action carried us through. And while the rebuild was daunting, as I will soon share, the following rituals helped me stay focused and radiate a powerful aura of joy, hope, and bliss during challenging times.

This week, we will address common momentum killers like distractions, perfectionism, setbacks, overwhelm, and boundaries. We will learn to say no in order to say yes to your soul's authentic desires.

Focus to Dissolve Distractions

You have to smell it. You have to hear it.
You have to feel it, everything.
—Emily Cook, Olympic freestyle skier

Focus helps us pay attention to what we authentically desire in the midst of distractions and setbacks. It also sustains the energy and momentum that's needed to reach our long-term visions. Without sustained focus, it's easy to get distracted by a lower vibration, lose our momentum and radiance, and lose sight of our higher goals.

What follows is an example of how blocking a distraction can work to your benefit. Let's talk hurtful gossip. I went through a challenging period many years ago when I learned through friends that a business colleague was gossiping about me behind my back, which was extremely painful. My dear friends, who were trying to protect me, wanted me to end it by addressing the issue head-on, but instead, I decided to let the gossiper shoot arrows, because I decided my ego would not be there. I would not gossip back, address it, or give it any energy. Instead, I bought a painting named *Silence* by the talented Iranian artist Kasra Namvari, whom I'd met at his gallery showing in downtown Manhattan. The vibrant artwork depicts a woman sitting on a tall, colorful ledge in a beautiful dress, silently reading a book of roses. The roses are falling from the pages and onto a glorious mound of red, orange, pink, and yellow roses on the ground. To me, this painting depicts how the woman's positive, flourishing energy can feed beauty and brilliance when focused desire is paired with inspired action.

As this business colleague continued to talk behind my back, I chose to meditate with this painting in front of me every morning, which inspired me to stay focused on what mattered for me and on the highest good of everyone else, too: my business and those who genuinely care about women's empowerment. If I had put my attention on the gossip, I would have diminished precious energy that could be fueling good things and would have lost any momentum gained from higher pursuits. I chose to stay focused on building a mission-driven company that values a talented team of authentic women who are making a huge impact in this world through our natural products, uplifting self-care messages, and charitable work. With laserlike focus, we have manifested facial peels, serums, masks, creams, and this book to help others nourish their own radiance.

Demi-intention creates demi-results. This ritual will give you the tools to rise above distractions in order to pour all of your focus into manifesting your beautiful roses.

RITUAL: Focus

To dissolve distractions

Time: 10–20 minutes

Ingredients: Pen and paper or a digital device

Optional Upgrades: Candle, crystals, a comfortable seat, essential oils

Notes: If desired, put one drop of peppermint oil on the palm of your hands and rub them together. Lightly cup your palms over your nose and mouth, breathing in and out until you feel centered and calm. You may want to have your Manifest Wheel and Radiance Intentions from week 7 as reference points. For this ritual, you can choose any of the following three options to help dissolve distractions for greater focus.

1. **Daydream.** Use your mind to play out a "movie" of you, as you live out your desire. Take your time and use four of your senses: see, hear, smell, and feel everything as if you are the star of this movie. As I've mentioned before, focus on how you want to *feel it,* above anything else, so that you can practice that vibration in your own movie.

2. **Visualize.** Create any visual on a vision board, in a book, in a journal, or on a Pinterest board to provide vivid color and inspiration. Use magazine clippings, photographs, or drawings with colorful felt pens. Seeing what you want (like my roses painting) creates a magnet and momentum between desire and reality; manifestation will come more quickly and easily.

3. **Listen.** Read out loud and record your Radiance Intentions on your cell phone and listen to them before going to sleep, first thing in the morning, before a meditation, or while walking. You will feel radiant from hearing your desires.

Prototype to Overcome Perfectionism

Nobody looks stupid when they're having fun.
—**Amy Poehler,** from *Yes Please*

One of the most popular concepts that I've taught women is how to create a "prototype" in order to overcome the inertia of perfectionism, a bona fide momentum killer. What does it mean to do this? A prototype is the tangible version of an idea that transforms what's in your imagination into something "real" that you can touch, see, or feel.

This can be an object, or it can encompass bigger experiences, iterations, and experiments that move you closer toward reaching a tangible goal or the kind of life that you wish to create for yourself.

People often ask me, "How did you create your creams?" and the honest answer is, I did it by prototyping. When I first created my creams in my kitchen as a hobby, my vision was simply to create luxurious products for my mom, sisters, and me, ones that weren't chock-full of chemical fillers. I lovingly chose each ingredient for its healing benefits and began experimenting in between practicing Mozart and Beethoven at the piano. My first concoction was a mixture of olive oil and sesame oil. It was too greasy, so I scoured library books and online articles to find what ingredient would make it less greasy. I added coconut oil and then shea butter. And so it went, day after day, until I made over one thousand prototypes of just one product. Each experiment was an opportunity to discover what worked and what didn't. The journey was a physically and spiritually healing process because, for once in my life, I was allowed to make mistakes. There were no outside pressures from an audience, critics, or teachers in my kitchen.

All goals and manifestations start with the vision, and all of your experiences that begin to turn this vision into reality are instrumental prototypes. These get better over time as you build momentum and move closer to your goal. When I finally landed on the first lotion that was worthy of bottling with a homemade label, that was my first prototype. I thought it was delightful because it was whipped, creamy, and smelled like lavender, but when my sister told me she thought it was too sticky and goopy, I had to take her feedback and apply it to the next batch. Dozens of prototypes later—as I evaluated, improved, and grew through the process—my final product eventually emerged.

In life, we often start strong with a project. Then, if it doesn't feel like a smashing success, we feel dejected and want to give up. But once you see some version of it in tangible form, build on that momentum, and create the next prototype, that brings your reality closer to what you envisioned.

An experience or prototype can be big or small: a blueprint for building a home, an outline for a business idea, or a new recipe. Anything that comes from your head and can be seen, touched, or felt is a "prototype." Your first prototype might be terrible, and know that it's completely fine. Most people allow perfectionism to kill the process, but this is where many fall short. They feel like they have failed and then stop. But when this happens, you have not failed. You just didn't maintain the momentum to continue on to the next prototype. The reason I love to use the word "prototype" is that, by definition, it is meant to be molded, tested, and experimented upon. It allows for mistakes, failures, and adjustments, which are often precursors to success.

RITUAL: Prototype

To overcome perfectionism or feeling stuck

Time: 5–15 minutes

Ingredients: Pen and paper or a digital device

Optional Upgrades: Candle, crystals, background music, flowers, cup of tea

Notes: This is a mindset ritual that helps you to overcome perfectionism.

1. **Breathe.** Close your eyes, breathing in and out until you feel deeply grounded in the present moment.
2. **Observe.** Examine and think about every aspect of your prototype. Did it reach the full potential that you had envisioned? If it didn't, consider the following:
   - What worked?
   - What didn't?
   - What shifts do I need to make for the next prototype?
     For example, while I was creating my lotions and potions, I would write, "Too sticky; use less butter for the next lotion."

3. **Intend.** Write down or note the steps you'd like to take and how you will proceed for the next round.

4. **Tune.** Check in to see how you are feeling about the process, and commit to how you'd like to feel during the next steps in order to radiate this feeling into your next prototype.

Resilience to Bounce Back

Barn's burnt down—now I can see the moon.
—**Mizuta Masahide, Japanese poet**

Resilience is the ability to bounce back after a setback, which is key to feeding momentum. When I think of resilience, I always think of New York City, a city that always comes back stronger in the face of adversity, such as the 9/11 attack and the COVID-19 pandemic.

When Governor Andrew Cuomo ordered a citywide lockdown during the pandemic, Savor Spas—along with all brick-and-mortars—were forced to temporarily close during a year of devastation and change. As the world tried to make sense of the chaos caused by record deaths and the violence against blacks and Asians, I could see the emotional toll that it took on my team. It was isolating to work from home without live camaraderie and community support.

What's more, the lure and enticement of Manhattan diminished with a lack of events, performances, and night-life. Many Manhattanites fled for greener, suburban pastures, and I watched stores and restaurants close and fold under the financial duress. I chose to stay in the city with my daughter, knowing that, because of its passion and creativity, this resilient town would not die. I witnessed a glimmer of hope when restaurants were allowed to open for outdoor seating in the freezing cold. A city that once had curb-to-curb traffic now erected heated cabins with firefly night-lights and winter greenery on the streets. It began to feel more like Paris than Manhattan, with a plethora of outdoor experiences: heated igloos with views of the city, and movie nights, magnificent free light shows, and rooftop cabins with blankets and fondue.

For me as a business owner, the prospect of bouncing back after such a huge setback was daunting. Over the past five years, we built a Savor Spa membership with hundreds of facial club members who'd be treated to a monthly facial. Within months of the closures, most of our members moved out of the city, and our membership dwindled to the double digits. We had painstakingly trained our select team of aestheticians, and then most moved back home or out of state to take care of family. I told my friends that it felt like we had built an intricate LEGO castle over years and, in an instant, it all fell to pieces.

At one point when I was feeling down about all this, my

friend Paul Merkelo (his inspiring story is in week 8) said to me, "Resilience is not a quick fix. It's slow and methodical, and more rational rather than emotional." I love this definition of resilience, because we often get stuck in the mire of feeling emotionally knocked down, but we can take great relief, replenishment, and renewal in good people, an elevated mindset, and baby steps toward normalcy. The following ritual will help you tap into your inner resources if you face a setback, in order to keep your momentum to reach radiant resilience.

RITUAL: Resilience

To come back after a setback

Time: 10–20 minutes

Ingredients: Pen and paper or a digital device

Optional Upgrades: Candle, crystals, background music, flowers, cup of tea

Notes: The Prototype and Resilience rituals have similar questions and aspects, but the latter addresses the spiritual and soul mindset. For instance, I used the Prototype ritual for making creams and leaned on the Resilience ritual to build the spas back up after COVID-19 closures.

1. **Observe.** When you feel knocked down from a setback, failure, or disappointment, become aware of *what* it is and *why* it is bringing you down.

2. **See.** The adage that goes, "Barn's burnt down— now I can see the moon" reminds us that clarity often rises from chaos.

   a. What is now clear to you? (Don't skip this question. It may take time but it is illuminating!)

   b. Are there lessons learned? If so, what are they?

   c. What is working and flowing for you?

   d. What will you commit to doing differently?

3. **Focus.** What is one small step you can take today to bounce back? This can become a "weed" that you pull or a "seed" that you plant tomorrow.

4. **Plan.** Carve out time to dedicate to this one step. If it is a challenge getting started, "hold the space" (see the week 8 ritual) for seven minutes to get the momentum started. Also, think of a friend, colleague, mentor, or loved one whom you can reach out to for support.

5. **Appreciate.** What are you grateful for?

6. **Affirm.** Say an affirmation, such as, *"I continually renew myself with grace and ease."* You can add this to your affirmations deck.

Organize Your Gorgeous Chaos

For every minute spent in organizing, an hour is earned.
—**Benjamin Franklin**

The term "gorgeous chaos" was first used when I had a friend visit me for a day a decade ago. She followed me around as I went to my West Village spa, had staff meetings, held a press interview, and then ran home to my then newborn to breastfeed her. My phone was buzzing and pinging the entire night, and at the end of the night over a glass of wine, she looked at me and said, "Your life is gorgeous chaos. So much chaos around you, but what emerges is that you focus on the gorgeousness of your life. I have no idea how you do it. I would drown in this."

One of the biggest blockers to momentum and radiance is overwhelm. Feeling overwhelmed can feel like you are drowning in a monsoon, and it's understandable if you want to stop all momentum to gain composure. Eventually, as I've mentioned before, this chronic busy-ness became unsustainable, but one skill that I learned during this time period was to stay focused on the "gorgeous" part of chaos by compartmentalizing for peace of mind.

I want to encourage you to think about your life as if it were one big household closet. Imagine opening a closet with zero structure: bed linens crumpled up, ponytail holders and bobby pins everywhere, expired makeup lurking in the back. Every time you open this closet, the chaos is draining. This is what our life energy can feel like if we don't structure our days to keep overwhelm (and stress wrinkles!) at bay. Think of the random items in the closet as tasks and to-dos. One of the kindest forms of self-care is to put those tasks into a container to organize them. Out of the chaos emerges gorgeous productivity, reducing anxiety and giving you a soothing structure. This becomes a support that helps you to flow with the momentum you've created.

You can organize your gorgeous chaos by batching together like ideas, thoughts, and tasks and putting them into project containers, just as you would in a well-organized closet. An example from the *Savor Beauty Planner*'s Organize Your "Gorgeous Chaos" section is shown below.

IV ORGANIZE YOUR "GORGEOUS CHAOS"
Extra Daily To-Do's, Notes, Meal Planning, Projects

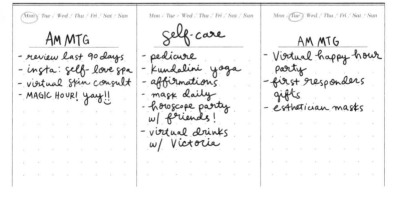

~~Mon~~ Tue / Wed / Thu / Fri / Sat / Sun	Mon / Tue / Wed / Thu / Fri / Sat / Sun	Mon / ~~Tue~~ / Wed / Thu / Fri / Sat / Sun
AM MTG	**self-care**	**AM MTG**
- review last 90 days	- pedicure	- Virtual happy hour party
- insta: self-love spa	- Kundalini yoga	- first responders gifts
- virtual skin consult	- affirmations	- esthetician masks
- MAGIC HOUR! yay!! ☺	- mask daily	
	- horoscope party w/ friends!	
	- virtual drinks w/ Victoria	

You also can create themed days to batch projects together, which gives your week a soothing rhythm and peace of mind. For example, here are my themed days:

MON	Money day! Pay bills, create weekly budget
TUE	Passion project day
WED	Wellness day: massage, pilates, green juice!
THU	Passion project day
FRI	Fun Fridays! Marketing, leave for country home
SAT	Social day: music lessons, dinner with friends
SUN	Self-care day: Savor Beauty planner time, blow-out, mask

The rhythmic structure for rituals and routines brings beauty and balance. Eventually many of the rituals in this book will become yours, and the following will help bake them into your week.

RITUAL: Organize Your "Gorgeous Chaos"

To shift from feeling undeserving to worthy

Time: 5–10 minutes

Ingredients: Journal and pen, a digital device, or the *Savor Beauty Planner*

Optional Upgrades: Candle, crystals, background music, flowers, cup of tea

Notes: Organize your time like a well-organized closet. Batch together like tasks and projects to stay organized and focused.

1. **Box.** Create four to six boxes in your planner or journal. Label each box with a project title. For example, I am in the process of finding summer camps for my daughter. I name that box "Summer Camps" and write down the camps I want to research.
2. **Batch.** Put all of the tasks together under each project. For each meeting, I think of everything I need to cover and list them. This keeps me feeling prepared and poised.
3. **Check.** As you accomplish each task, make sure to check it off for a happy endorphin hit!

4. Appreciate. State aloud what you are grateful for. For example:

"I appreciate feeling organized and peaceful."

Boundaries

You need boundaries. . . . Even in our material creation, . . .
boundaries mark the most beautiful of places, between
the ocean and the shore, between the mountains and
the plains, where the canyon meets the river.

—Wm. Paul Young, Canadian author

One of the most important ways to increase and maintain momentum is to protect your energy. And nothing dissipates precious energy more than going against your authentic desires, goals, or needs. Creating boundaries is honoring the inner voice that says not to sacrifice your needs to please another. It also is an invisible force field that allows you to own what is yours and let go of what isn't. This is different from selfishness and doesn't mean we disregard what others want or abandon responsibilities; it simply means that if mutual desires are not in harmony for the greater good, we say no to that which does not serve us in order to say yes to that which does.

When the 2021 #stopasianhate movement heated up, I received numerous requests from the press to speak about my experiences and point of view. Growing up in a pre-dominantly white community in Iowa, microaggressions and stereotyping were daily occurrences. I saw my dad's broken English taunted, and my sisters and I were bullied for the shape of our eyes. My parents insisted that we ignore the racist comments and rise above them by working hard to succeed.

During this recent spate of violence against Asians, I sadly reacted by thinking, "Well, nothing from my childhood has changed." My friend Mona, who is a successful Asian entrepreneur and creative, decided to fuel her anger by scripting a monologue play. We began talking about the sexual harassment of Asian women, so that she would have fodder to consider for her important piece. I shared with her how common it was for me to get racially catcalled on the streets with comments like, "Hey, China girl, *arigato!*" The men would do this while pressing their hands together in a subservient bow. As I told Mona, "It's insulting on so many levels. First, I'm Korean, not Chinese or Japanese. And then there are the racialized sexual overtones. . . . I used to feel so embarrassed, like I did something wrong, so I would cross the street to avoid them."

Mona loved the message and asked me to record it for her monologue. I immediately agreed. Yet when a few days passed, I couldn't seem to do it. I agonized over this decision. I wanted to support Mona, but I didn't feel ready to speak about the harassment. I needed more time to process.

I felt torn about what to do, because I did not want to say no to my friend Mona and to such an important cause.

I finally realized that moving forward with an energy of hesitancy was detrimental to both of us. I was not honoring my authentic desire, and it was not fair to Mona to approach her project with indecision. She needed fire and passion, not ambivalence and delay. I sent her a text that said:

> Mona, love, I really don't feel comfortable doing this. I adore you to bits and pieces, so I wanted to do this for you, but I'm not feeling authentic about it. I hope you understand.

By setting healthy boundaries, we prioritize our feelings and desires so we can protect our energy field to create flow and momentum. Mona's immediate response was:

> Totally understand! I'll sort it out—thank you!

All the drama I'd built up in my head was self-imposed; Mona was fine, and we had dinner with our significant others a month later. If you are having a hard time with boundaries, the following ritual will help clarify and articulate a kind no.

RITUAL: Healthy Boundaries

To gain clarity around boundaries

Time: 5–10 minutes

Ingredients: Pen and paper or a digital device

Optional Upgrades: Soothing music, crystals, honey face mask, warm moist towel

Notes: I like to do this ritual with a honey face mask to create a purifying environment and soothing space for clarity. You can use a manuka-honey face mask or easily make your own from items in your kitchen pantry. I love manuka honey for the detoxifying and healing enzymes that draw impurities from the skin. Mix two teaspoons of organic honey with one teaspoon oil (I prefer safflower oil, used by Korean women as far back as AD 918, for a lightweight glossy sheen), and add one drop of lavender essential oil.

1. **Mask.** Apply the soothing honey mask onto cleansed, moist skin in upward motions to purify and clarify the skin. At any point during this ritual, if your skin begins to tingle, you can gently remove the mask with a warm moist towel and apply a hydrating cream to provide a finishing nourishing treatment.

2. **Breathe.** Breathe in and out while drawing your awareness to your shoulders, neck, and jaw. Allow each breath to release any tension until you feel focused, relaxed, and clear.

3. **Ask.** Reflect on the following questions as they relate to your situation:

   a. What is the situation at hand?

   b. Are my needs, goals, and desires being honored?

   c. If not, why am I not honoring them?

4. **Meditate.** You can meditate to clear the mind, or you can also do the Higher Self meditation (from week 3) to access higher levels of clarity.

5. **Write.** If you want to say no to someone, craft a response that you feel good about. Here are some gracious statements:

   - I'm honored but I can't.
   - I wish there were two of me!
   - I want to give this my all, and I just can't right now.
   - My plate is full right now.
   - No, thank you, but it sounds lovely, so perhaps next time.
   - I'm not taking on anything else right now.

6. **Affirm.** Create an affirmation around boundaries, such as, *"By saying no I'm saying yes to what's important to me."* Make sure to add this to your affirmations deck.

Your Momentum Plan

1. **Customize.** Decide which rituals will support you this week. My suggestion is to try them all as you need them and then ritualize those that resonate.
   - FOCUS (to dissolve distractions)
   - PROTOTYPE (to overcome perfectionism or feeling stuck)
   - RESILIENCE (to come back after a setback)
   - ORGANIZE YOUR "GORGEOUS CHAOS" (to handle overwhelm)
   - HEALTHY BOUNDARIES (to gain clarity around boundaries)
2. **Plan.** Write in your planner or put in a GCal reminder when you will do these rituals. Remember that scheduling in rituals prioritizes *you*!
3. **Cleanse.** Don't forget to cleanse and moisturize your skin at night while saying your affirmations!
4. **Affirm.** Create three to five self-worth affirmations. Write them on sticky notes, in your journal, or add to your affirmations deck. For example:
   "I bounce back with resilience and beauty."
5. **Love.** Schedule a self-love activity that elevates your flow.

SAVOR ABUNDANCE

When most people hear the term "abundance," they assume that it means "having" or "accumulating" everything they need or crave. But it's so much deeper than that. Abundance is actually about living in the ethos of "being, doing, and receiving." Abiding by this mindset is what allows the floodgates of a truly rich and prosperous life to open.

Let's break this down. "Being" abundant means feeling whole and complete. "Doing" abundantly is about holding space every day for inspired action. "Receiving" abundance is about welcoming gifts with open arms, even if it's not exactly what we expected because the universe delivers in mysterious and glorious ways. The result is an ability to embody true abundance, which allows us to then radiate an aura of confidence and ease since we have all the love, self-worth, well-being, time, money, energy, and resources that we desire. We also inspire others because our cup overflows with a replenishing energy that's truly irresistible and attractive.

Together, we are going to increase the good things in your life, and this begins with feeling grateful for what we have now. How we go about being energetically present, appreciating what we already have, and then opening ourselves up to receive more can usher in prosperity's flow. The best part? It's completely free to tune in to this vibration of richness and opportunity. The more we can approach life—from mundane to monumental moments—with an attitude of gratitude, the more we will radiate abundance, which then attracts more abundance.

Being able to navigate your way through trials and yet come out on top is another example of "gorgeous chaos." When things get chaotic, stressful, or negative, there is always a gorgeous gift that emerges if you take the time to see it and savor the beauty. A scarcity mindset is one that resists the present by trying to alter, judge, control, criticize, or manipulate versus one that appreciates and allows each moment's beauty to emerge.

One of my best friends, Sara, was going through a rough time with her boyfriend of three years. One night around dinnertime, she realized she only had leftover waffles and bacon in the fridge to serve her son. She called it a "mom fail," but made it anyway. This made her eleven-year-old son groan. "How gross, Mom! I'm *not* eating that!" And instead of trying to hide her feelings in the moment, Sara gave into, and sat with them . . . in tears.

"Honey, I'm having a hard day and can't make anything

else right now," she explained. "I need you to be under-standing and just eat this for tonight." That's when Sara's "gorgeous" emerged from the chaos: her loving son gave her a big, squishy hug. "Are you okay, Mom?" he asked. "Don't worry, I have your back." His support was a gift, and an abundant one at that.

So we serve a less-than-desirable meal, deal with disappointing news, or listen to upset loved ones, and we experience lack or loss if we choose to remain stuck in these moments. The alternative is to take Sara's approach: accept what's happening around you without judgment, sit with the honesty of it, and remain open to the gorgeous that's bound to emerge. That's when we receive gratitude, lessons, joy, support, and love—the hallmarks of abundance.

Creating an Abundance Mindset

For beautiful eyes, look for the good in others; for beautiful lips, speak only words of kindness; and for poise, walk with the knowledge that you are never alone.

—Audrey Hepburn

One of my favorite sayings is the one by Audrey Hepburn just quoted. So much beauty comes from within us, and when we see goodness in all of life's possibilities and reflect that on the outside, abundance is sure to follow.

The universe honors this and guides us toward a life that matches these high-vibrational intentions.

Creating an abundance mindset requires believing that there are always opportunities for vibrant growth; we see a world full of plenty, and fortuity is always within reach. There is no room for jealousy or envy, since we're deeply aware that there is ample abundance for everyone. In fact, when your soul feels expansive and rich, you will see others' possessions and successes as proof that there's enough to go around.

Abundance nourishes us when we can balance all three parts of "being, doing, and receiving." Traci Bild, a talented entrepreneur, friend, and client who participated in my manifesting programs, has amassed financial wealth as a businesswoman. She recently moved into her astounding dream home in Florida, which she and her husband built over five arduous years. It wasn't an easy road, though. Over half a decade, I watched Traci handle the grueling details involved in the process of buying land, negotiating with contractors, and working with her design team. When our friends finally celebrated her home's beautiful completion, I had chills all over my body as she gave us a tour. It was stunning, and every themed room reflected her heart. After the tour, Traci reminded us that she'd once lived in a trailer as a child. She had come so far and achieved so much in life—and all because she'd deeply learned to claim, groom, and embody an energetically abundant frame of mind.

"Ladies, this dream home symbolizes that abundance and wealth is a state of being," she said. "A few months ago, I felt down because of a lot of chaos: my kids needed me, the home rebuild was stalling due to complications, and my business was doing well but not meeting our financial goals. So the first thing I always do whenever I'm in that discombobulated state is to *protect my mind*; it's so important to be fiercely protective of what we let into our headspace.

"I distinctly remember one afternoon during this period that was pivotal for me," she continued.

I made myself an espresso and pulled out my vision board to reset my mindset of possibility. I went back to what's important to me, like getting my daughter ready for high school graduation, helping my son launch his summer business, focusing on my health, and making our new home beautiful and magical with pretty gardens. I said to the universe, "I don't want a fish. I want a whale." What I meant was that I wanted to be in the abundance mindset, not one of scarcity. I said it with conviction and passion, and I *expected* it. I started to regain confidence and continued to do what I do daily: I got on the phone and made sales calls. Well, guess what? At 3 P.M. a whale arrived. A huge, ripe opportunity landed in my inbox, and it confirmed what I know about abundance. When I'm doing my part, the universe partners with me every single time.

You can see from Traci's story that she embodies the abundance mindset of "being, doing, and receiving." When the chips were down, she shifted from a scarcity to abundance mindset, simply by reminding herself of who she is and what she wants out of life. And she did her part, too, by putting in the work to see her goals to completion. Sure enough, that's when Traci received her "whale," from partnering with the universe. Staying in this mode is no easy feat. This next ritual will help you reset possibilities and progress to be radiantly abundant, too.

RITUAL: Abundance Mindset

To shift from a mindset of lack to abundance

Time: 15–30 minutes

Ingredients: Pen and paper or a digital device

Optional Upgrades: Candles, crystals, fresh rose or other flower

Notes: You can simply reflect on these thought starters or you can write them down and journal.

1. **Be.** Breathe in four seconds. If you have a rose, inhale the beautiful aroma as a symbol of abundance. Hold for five seconds.

Breathe out. Repeat until you can feel grounded.

2. Do. Pull out your Manifest Wheel, Radiance Intentions, or a visual that inspires you. Ask yourself if you are doing your part so that the universe can partner with you. If the answer is yes, affirm that when you receive the abundance, the timing will be perfect. If no, reflect on what seeds you could be planting and then commit to holding the space (from week 8, "Grow Little by Little").

3. Receive. Ask yourself, "What's gorgeous in the chaos?" Allow the subsequent gifts to flow into your life by focusing on plenty and progress versus the lack of what you have. Write down the lessons you are learning.

Time Abundance

Once she stopped rushing through life, she was amazed
by how much more life she had time for.
—Unknown

One of the most precious commodities we have is time, and unlike financial abundance, time is irreplaceable. Once time passes us by, it's gone.

As a concert pianist, I learned that we can stretch time with a simple little trick. On a less-than-optimal performance night, I would feel hurried and rushed onstage, like time was cut in half and I was scrambling to the finish line. On the best of nights, however, I felt like I could magically stretch time. I felt like an eagle, entirely in control and poised, with all the time in the world to envelop the audience with sound, rhythm, and emotion. The former scenario felt desperate and panicked; the latter felt succulent and rich.

The secret for time expansion? Feel as grounded as possible. No matter how anxious and rushed I felt, the antidote was always the same: I'd center myself by allowing my breath to naturally rise and fall, and then feel my body relax into the earth. My shoulders would drop a few inches, as the muscles in my jaw and neck instantly melted. Before a performance, I took as much time as I needed to feel calm and at peace before walking on stage. I did everything I could to be in the moment and feel gratitude for the path that led me there. I'd feel my footsteps tap the ground, listen to the applause, bow slowly, look those in the audience in their eyes, and express silent gratitude toward them.

By staying grounded, I'd let go of the past and the future and become fully immersed in the present. This would always open the door to the unexpected gift of time. Instead of feeling panicked and rushed, I'd center myself and assume the mindset of someone who has an abundance of time. Where I always landed was what I call "my sweet spot," a place where I can appreciate both enjoyable and challenging moments because I'd created mental space for it.

Today, I still practice this art of expanding time in my daily life. A typical day for me can feel rushed and hurried as I get my daughter ready for school, walk the dog, make breakfast, attend work meetings, cook dinner, and spend quality time with my partner. Wearing the many hats of mom, career woman, and lover makes me feel fulfilled and complete, but sometimes with so much going on, my mind experiences a "traffic jam," with too many thoughts crossing simultaneously. I'm sure you can relate. So when I begin to feel a deficit of time, all I have to do is look for my sweet spot, which the following ritual will help you to do, too!

RITUAL: Time Abundance
To find your sweet spot through time expansion

Time: 1+ minute
Notes: This is a ritual that you can lean into at any moment of the day when you feel rushed and want to ground yourself for time abundance.

1. **Inhale.** Put one hand on your lower belly and feel it expand as you take in a big breath.

2. **Exhale.** Allow your belly to decompress like an accordion as you breathe out.

3. **Relax.** Keep your inner attention on the rhythm of this breath as you imagine your body staying grounded and relaxed. Feel your feet on the floor. Take in what's before you by seeing, listening, and feeling.

4. **Be.** Wherever you are, be all there. Choose to focus on one thing at a time. Trust that the universe is taking care of anything that is not in your immediate control right now.

5. **Reduce.** Consider reducing the amount of work or commitments you have during the day and giving yourself a little more space and grace to be fully present.

6. **Affirm.** Whenever you feel rushed for time, choose an affirmation that anchors you, such as, *"I am grounded and present"* or *"I have time abundance."*

7. **Replenish.** Inevitably, time will become rushed as you dive into your day. Replenish your time abundance by repeating this ritual over and over again.

Resource Abundance

You can't be a resource for others unless you nourish yourself.
—**Alexandra Stoddard, author**

When I was building my business, I didn't have funding from investors or family. Instead, I leaned on the belief that creativity was my million-dollar ticket. Instead of telling myself, "I can't do this" or "I can't afford it," I'd ask myself, "How can I do this and how can I afford it?" Then I'd get creative with resources, ideas, and solutions to solve any given challenge. During my company's early build, it would have been easy to buy into a scarcity mindset by focusing on what I didn't have and was losing, especially when my bank account would drop lower than I was comfortable with. However, my abundance mindset inspired me to instead focus on progress and what's available, knowing that there were plenty of resources to help me.

When I opened the first Savor Beauty brick-and-mortar store, I had to find creative solutions and resources to get us up and running. To secure a space in Manhattan's celebrity-studded West Village neighborhood, landlords require up to six months for a security deposit, which was a six-figure amount that I didn't have in the bank. So instead, I scoured Craigslist, an online classified site, for other options and found a sweet little shop being sublet by an artist. She wanted out of the lease and was willing to be flexible with the rent and security deposit. I offered $12,000 for the security deposit, to which the artist agreed, and this was the beginning of Savor Beauty + Spa.

Think of abundant resources as experts, ideas, perspectives, and tools that will help you grow, improve, and elevate any possible goal that you might have in mind. Here are some examples of resources that I tap into whenever I want a solution to a challenge:

- Healers for self-care
- Doctors for physical well-being
- Therapists for mental health
- Friends and family for fun and love
- Colleagues for referrals and solutions
- Mentors for growth ideas
- Google for research
- Teachers for learning new skills
- Airbnb for travel and experiences
- Books for solutions
- Coaches for positive growth
- Online services for matching to pros and like-minded people
- Apps for making life easier and more interesting
- Google maps for restaurants, stores, and more

- YouTube for learning anything and everything
- Social media for discovering and deepening hobbies

The list can go on and on, but the vital thing to remember is that whenever you feel a need, void, or are stuck, there is an abundance of resources and solutions to help and elevate you.

RITUAL: Resource Abundance

To find solutions, tools, and ideas to solve a challenge

Time: 10+ minutes
Ingredients: Pen and paper or a digital device
Optional Upgrades: Background music, candles, crystals, eye cream
Notes: This is a ritual you can do whenever you feel stuck or need a solution to a pain point.

1. **Nourish.** Apply an eye cream to renew the skin, as a symbol that you will be seeing and discovering new resources. Place three dots around your eyes and lightly pat the cream in. I like to gently "play the piano" around my eyes to give it a light stimulation

while allowing the nutrients to absorb into the delicate skin.

2. Clarify. Think of a current pain point or challenge that you're having and clarify what you want. You can write it out if it helps you, for example: "I want to sell my apartment and want to find an excellent real estate agent."

3. Affirm. Say an affirmation like, *"There are plenty of options in the world."* Saying any phrase that begins with *"There are plenty of . . ."* illuminates abundance.

4. Strategize. Think of ideas, resources, and solutions. Asking others for ideas or referrals is a great way to think outside the box.

5. Outreach. Plant seeds by contacting people, looking up resources, and finding solutions.

6. Appreciate. Once you find a solution that works for you, savor the abundance you've tapped into!

Space Abundance

There are two ways to be rich: One is by acquiring much, and the other is by desiring little.

—Jackie French Koller, author

My mom and I could not be more different in one way: she is a self-proclaimed accumulator, and I am a die-hard minimalist. Growing up, my mom delighted in collecting every "free gift with purchase" from all the cosmetic brands at our local mall. Her bathroom closet was packed with countless cream and lipstick samples, and her vanity was cluttered with empty jars and tubes. When I would come home from college, she often asked me to help her clean out her closets. I'd spend hours purging and organizing, and even though she protested whenever I suggested she throw some of her items in the trash bag, I'd later hear her on the phone, bragging to her sisters that I'd helped her out and that she could breathe better with more space. And then, of course, she'd hint, "I have more space, so you can send me the best new cream in Seoul!"

It elevates our vibration and helps us to breathe easier when we've cleared our own space of things we no longer value or use. I believe that people and things all have an energetic force, and we should love and/or use what we own. In fact, there's a concept called "animism," which is the belief that objects, places, creatures, and even words each possess a soul and a distinct spiritual essence that is animated and alive. My rule of thumb is that if something doesn't uplift my energy or if I haven't used it in one year—provided that it isn't of sentimental value—it should not take up precious space.

To this point, I have a ritual of cleaning out my wardrobe, pantries, and closets, which gives me mental room to breathe more freely. I choose one area to focus on for just seven minutes and create an intention to have space abundance. I take a recycle and trash bag in one hand, a giveaway bag in the other, and I begin to purge. I'm purposeful about what I want to keep or what has expired and needs to move on. This ritual also helps me take inventory of what I have. For example, in the process of clearing my wardrobe for refreshed energy, I inevitably find a pretty dress and fancy shoes that I have forgotten about. Or, when I clean out and organize my spice pantry, I see what spices I do have, which inspires new cooking recipes. Finding and enjoying these things is celebrating abundance, an unexpected gift of clearing the space.

This next ritual will help you clear space for more abundant energy to flow into your life.

RITUAL: Space Abundance

To love and value what you own

Time: 7+ minutes weekly

Ingredients: Bags to recycle, trash, and give items away

Optional Upgrades: Upbeat music

Notes: I like to do this ritual weekly and focus on one targeted area, like a pantry or closet drawer.

1. **Choose.** Identify which area of your home you will clear out. Choose one that is small and manageable. You will feel accomplished when you take on a smaller space versus potentially feeling overwhelmed by trying to conquer a large room.

2. **Time.** Set the timer for seven minutes. At the end of seven minutes, you can stop—or keep going if you're on a roll!

3. **Clear.** When you begin the purging process, ask yourself these questions: "Do I love it? Is it of sentimental value? Will I need it for the occasional event or situation? Did I use it in the last year?" If the answer is no to all four, then toss the item(s) or give it (them) away.

4. **Purge.** Throw, recycle, or give away all the items you don't want or need.

5. **Appreciate.** Commit to valuing and using what you own or appreciating your newfound space!

"Sunny Day" Abundance

For those of us learning the way to financial serenity and
solvency, the envelope system teaches prudence, patience,
and perseverance. . . . You can only spend what you have.
—Sarah Ban Breathnach, **author**

One of the best money lessons I've ever learned was from my dad. I used to receive a weekly allowance from him for doing household chores. At the end of each week, he'd tell me to put 50 percent of my earnings into a piggy bank. Learning discipline like this at a young age taught me that only a portion of my earnings was ever available for spending. Sure enough, I still have this mindset today. It's allowed me to save for fun things like vacationing in Hawaii, for buying a home in Manhattan, and for splurging on a guilty pleasure, like a coveted designer purse.

Everyone talks about saving for a rainy day or retirement (both are very important), but no one talks about saving for a sunny day. Why is that? Isn't it just as essential to save for things that we can't wait to experience? Think about what it says to our soul, mind, and spirit to put so much energy into saving for something that could go wrong or when we retire versus saving for something that we get to celebrate and savor. Intending to create a "Sunny Day Fund" opens up the channel to receive more abundance, fun, and laughter.

We all love blissful experiences: going on vacation, buying our favorite things, enjoying a spa day. Splurging and savoring something with cheerful abandon is revitalizing and refreshing. However, we often feel guilty in the process because we overspend, and the beautiful feelings associated with the experience are sabotaged with negative associations. The overriding sentiment becomes "I don't deserve this" or "I can't afford it." And then we stop giving ourselves these restorative moments in life because money guilt blocks our sunny bliss.

In week 2, we created your Radiance Retreats list, and now I'd like you to open a Sunny Day Fund to save for some of these pleasures. With this fund, you will spend responsibly (without going into debt) and 100 percent guilt-free. Over the years, I have used my Sunny Day Fund to take a candle workshop, fly to Paris, or buy a beautiful piece of jewelry. The amazing deal with this fund is that you can spend the cash as lavishly and abundantly as you wish. No one gets to judge or dictate what you do with these savings. You've earned it, you deserve it, and you get to savor it. And while you're at it, you'll be exercising and strengthening your abundance muscles.

As a rule, I set aside around 5 percent of my paycheck for a sunny day. If you can only afford to do 1 percent, that's fine, too. What's important is to make this a ritual, so that you are consistently building abundance. If you have extra money coming in, set aside more. You will feel rejuvenated when you get to experience a treat that's been paid for exclusively by your Sunny Day Fund.

Sometimes it's essential to take certain leaps before you're ready. When I wanted to spend the summer in France, I knew that I had to purchase the plane tickets before getting nervous about leaving work for that long. Make the commitment and watch the magic unfold. Leap and the net will appear, as they say.

RITUAL: Sunny Day Fund
To increase your abundance mindset

Time: 30 minutes
Ingredients: Bank, paycheck
Optional Upgrades: Candle, crystals, beauty altar

1. **Open.** Go online and create a separate account to put aside 1–5 percent from every paycheck. Call it a Sunny Day Fund so that you can remind yourself that it's an investment in you.

2. **Choose.** Choose an experience that you want to savor. Refer to your Radiance Retreats and figure out which one you want to work toward. Consider how much it costs, and watch your fund grow as you put aside money. You can choose multiple goals,

but it's always fun to know exactly what you will get to savor as a result of your hard work.

3. **Percolate.** If you plan for a dream vacation, start gathering clips from newspapers and magazines of where you want to go, stay, and eat. Or, if you plan to purchase a fabulous pair of shoes, cut out a photo of them and put it into your vision book or on a vision board.

4. **Share.** Tell a trusted friend or loved one about this exciting project. There's nothing like getting friends, family, and a support group behind your mission to nourish your radiance.

5. **Affirm.** Every time you deposit into or spend money from your Sunny Day Fund, say an affirmation like, *"I am abundant and rich in all ways"* or *"I am fortunate to savor this experience, and I deserve it!"*

Your Abundance Plan

1. **Customize.** Pick and choose which rituals you will do this week.

   - ABUNDANCE MINDSET (to shift from lack to an abundance mindset)
   - TIME ABUNDANCE (to expand time by being fully present)
   - RESOURCE ABUNDANCE (to find solutions to relieve a pain point)

- SPACE ABUNDANCE (to love and value what you own)
- SUNNY DAY FUND (to increase your abundance mindset)

2. **Plan.** Write in your planner or put in a GCal reminder when you will do these rituals. Remember that scheduling in rituals prioritizes *you*!

3. **Cleanse.** Don't forget to cleanse and hydrate your skin at night while saying your affirmations!

4. **Affirm.** Create three to five self-worth affirmations. Write them on sticky notes, in your journal, or add to your affirmations deck, for example:

   "I am abundant and rich in all ways."

5. **Love.** Schedule a self-love activity that elevates your abundance.

GIVE, GIVE, GET

f I could invent the ultimate elixir that yielded pure radiance and glow, it would be named after my personal philosophy called, "Give, Give, Get." Give, Give, Get offers an abundance of opportunities to nourish like-minded, kindred spirits in your life (and in turn, you!)—and it has never let me down as a modus operandi. Practicing Give, Give, Get helps you to authentically invest in your relationships, which nurtures seamless connectedness and sustenance with others.

How we give is paramount, here. We can give from full or empty cups, but they each lead to very different outcomes. Before we delve deeper into this idea, let me first illustrate what it means to give, by sharing both the tragic and beautiful memories we gained after a family loss. This occurred when Chantal, the sister of my ex-husband, Marc, passed away from a sudden and very tragic accident, when she was just in her forties. Marc and I experienced the heart of her giving, when we traveled to Geneva to help his parents clean out her apartment and prepare for her wake.

Chantal was a collector of handbags, knickknacks, and all sorts of cute, artsy items; her eclectic treasures, however, were now her parents' burden, as they tried to sort through her belongings and decide what to do with them. We spent a full day tossing, recycling, and giving away most of her valuable possessions. That same evening, we hosted the wake. We asked her friends and coworkers to share a memory of Chantal. One friend told the story of how she always gave him Swiss chocolates when he was feeling down. Another recollected getting her hair done on a rainy day and how Chantal had given her an umbrella to protect her new do, even though this meant that Chantal would get wet. The overall mood at Chantal's wake was light and cheerful, and her parents felt proud of their daughter, as they heard stories about her generosity.

At the end of the day, I thought about how we work so hard during our lives to gain success and accumulate "things," but true value comes from the moments that we give of ourselves and how we make others feel. What lived on was not Chantal's many possessions but her generosity of spirit. What she gave to the world in those stories was essentially what I'd refer to as her "Gives," and they infused healing and renewal in everyone at the wake. Chantal is a perfect example of someone who gave from a cup full of generosity and authenticity.

So why are there two "Gives" in Give, Give, Get? Because when we give from a cup that overflows, our inner universe is so rich that we have an abundance of love, support, and connection to give generously. And what we get in return can range from good karma to feel-good vibes. A "Get" might happen if you donate to a charity and feel immense pleasure from it, or if you help a friend move and find that an hour later, a stranger randomly buys you coffee for no reason. You might even put in extra hours at work and get a surprise bonus, or give selflessly to your child and get a hug in return. These are all examples of boundless "Gets" in Give, Give, Get.

This entire book has been dedicated to how to fill your cup—aka how to fill your life with radiant, positive, and vibration-raising thoughts and experiences. When your cup is whole and full, you attract effervescent bonds that renew and revive your spirit. Those who give from a full cup also manage to do so while prioritizing their self-worth, self-care, and self-love so that they stay at a high frequency. If you constantly replenish self-love from rituals in this book, you can give authentically, meaning that you will give what you have and what you *want* to give. On the other hand, giving from an empty cup means doing it for approval or expecting something in return. Empty cuppers often give due to a lack of self-worth and self-love, and this scarcity energy is often returned to them.

Before I began intentionally nourishing my radiance and self-love, I often gave from an empty cup, one filled with the energy of lack. As a result, I would attract people into my life who used me for jobs, connections, and other ulterior motives. After a chain of disappointing interactions, I realized that I was the common denominator in this recurring pattern: my empty cup attracted others with empty cups.

There is a saying: "Nothing changes if nothing changes." So when I began practicing self-love rituals, I made it a point to start giving from a place of self-love and respect. And sure enough, I became a lighthouse that attracted other full-cuppers. Now I know that my dear, like-minded friends are just a text away from a soulful conversation that is an oasis of peace and fun. My partner and I can create meaningful time together and host fun dinner gatherings, dance parties, and travel getaways. We give (and get) laughter, meaningful conversation, delicious food, and fun times with friends and family about whom we deeply care.

Chellie Campbell, the author of one of my favorite books, *The Wealthy Spirit*, refers to choosing to spend time with full- and empty-cuppers as deciding whether to swim with dolphins or sharks. Simply put, dolphins are your people: they want the best for you, and you want the best for them. And after playing with fellow dolphins, you feel happy, peaceful, and playful. Then there are the sharks. Not surprisingly, sharks don't have your best interests in mind: they basically eat dolphins. After playing with sharks, you can feel wounded, betrayed, and empty.

Creating an inner circle of trusted, lifetime relationships—brimming with full-cuppers and dolphins, of course—comes from interactions with other givers who offer the meaningful and generous mutual support that we all desire so that we feel relationship joy.

Give Listening

I speak with the eyes, I listen with the heart,
I understand with time.

—French poetry

Listen with your ears. *Hear without the need to defend.*
Listen with your eyes. *See when the eyes light up or when the body closes.*
Listen with your mind. *Observe without judgment.*
Listen with your heart. *Feel and empathize with others.*
Listen with your skin. *Allow goose bumps to guide you.*
Listen with your guts. *Let intuition lead the way.*

The act of listening enriches our relationships and deepens our connections, which fortifies and enhances our Give, Give, Get practice. A 2003 study conducted by York University psychologist Faye Doell found that there are two different types of listening: listening to understand and listening to respond. The most healing balm that we can give to others is the gift of feeling heard and understood, and one of the best ways to do this is to listen with our eyes, even while we are speaking. I call this looking for the "light and linger" in others—i.e., if your listener's eyes light up, then you know that what you are saying matters to that person. If his or her eyes linger (looking to the side to process thought), then they may want to hear you say more or contribute to the conversation themselves. These cues allow for a more meaningful exchange.

When we conduct press meetings at Savor Beauty + Spa, listening with my eyes is the skill that helps me to connect most with magazine and online editors. Years ago, I had just been featured in *The New York Times* alongside Gwyneth Paltrow and Kate Hudson about the growing pubic-hair trend (no pun intended). It was circa 2013 when Paltrow mentioned on a talk show that she'd let her hair-down-there grow out. Since Savor Beauty + Spa once offered Brazilian waxing, *The Times* called me for a quote about this trend. (My nugget?: "Our clients in particular are eco- and health-minded, and the grown look certainly suits a girl who is more au naturel.")

After the article came out, producers from the *Today* show, *The Howard Stern Show*, and all the major magazines began to call for even more exclusive quotes and thoughts about this hairy subject. While the publicity would have been terrific for the company, I decided to turn all these outlets down because I didn't want to become known as the "pubic-hair expert." Savor Beauty's mission was about all things face, and I wanted to stay focused on our core mission.

Hannah, an editor, was working at a major national magazine around this time. She asked to visit me in the spa for an interview. I quickly realized that she, too, wanted a quote on pubic hair for a waxing story she was writing. As the interview progressed, I pivoted to the subject of Savor Beauty's Dollars & Scents program, in which we hire moms who are transitioning back into the workforce after raising children. Hannah's eyes instantly lit up. When I noticed this, I slowed down to allow her to ask me more questions, and the conversation flowed naturally. Anytime her eyes lingered to the side to process a thought, I paused to allow her to guide the conversation further.

Because I caught Hannah's important body-language cues by being an active listener, my "Get" was major: she ultimately dedicated an exclusive, full-page story in her high-profile magazine about Savor's origin story and how we enjoy giving back philanthropically.

This weekend, when you're with friends for coffee or having dinner with family, practice listening with your eyes. Once you notice the "light or linger" in your audience's gaze, you will know to feed a depth and dimension to your conversations that you might have otherwise missed.

RITUAL: Listen with Your Eyes

To connect with others on a meaningful level

Time: 10 minutes

Ingredients: Your eyes and a conversation

Notes: This ritual can be performed whenever you have a gathering of one or more people!

1. **Breathe.** Stay present and grounded throughout the conversation by noticing how you're breathing in and out.

2. **Awaken.** Become aware of the other person's eyes while you speak. If you notice the person's eyes glimmer or body open up, you will know that what you are talking about matters to the other person. They may even pipe in with a comment. You may have missed this cue in the past, but now you have greater awareness while you speak.

3. **Pause.** If the person's eyes linger to the side to process a thought, slow down and allow the other person to speak and ask questions. This will lead to a more meaningful connection.

4. **Flow.** Stay curious, interested, and engaged. After all, there's nothing more refreshing than getting out

of your head and expanding your world through another person's lens.

Give What Matters

It is not what we have that matters; what matters is what we give away with love.
—**Dr. Debasish Mridha, physician and philosopher**

When we authentically give what truly matters to someone in a relationship, the effort becomes a source of synergy and harmony. This is why I really appreciate the book *The 5 Love Languages* by Gary Chapman, because it teaches us how to give exactly what matters to our loved ones. The primary love languages that Chapman highlights are:

- Receiving gifts
- Quality time
- Acts of service
- Words of affirmation
- Physical touch

Through our means of love communication, we become aware of how another person expresses and receives love for richer dimensions of connection. Sometimes, even with the best intentions, we give it our all but the other person may not be able to receive it. For example, if one partner's love language is acts of service and the other's is physical touch, the former can give by cooking dinner every day but what matters to the other is to hold hands on a walk. Both have lovely intentions, but they miss the mark on giving what matters to the loved one.

The beauty of discovering what truly moves and impacts our counterparts is that we begin to understand what is of utmost importance to them. What's more, we can take this concept of love languages and apply it to every relationship that we have. For instance, I have a friend who sends me many texts of support. She's the friend who affirms my value every single time we talk. However, quality time is not as important to her. She prefers staying at home to nest over going out for a night on the town. At first, I felt rejected every time I'd ask her to go out, but I began to realize and appreciate that her forte isn't partying; it's support and wisdom.

I have another friend who loves quality time with her loved ones. A few years ago, I had planned to visit her in Colorado, and at the last minute, I felt stressed about work and leaving my daughter. When I called her to postpone, she became understandably upset and put her foot down. "Angela, our time together means the world to me," she said. "I've planned for it, and it will be upsetting if you back out now." She was absolutely right. I took the next flight out the following day, and together we bonded over spa days, rosé cocktails, and tarot-card readings. Giving what matters to my best friends has contributed to long-lasting and fruitful relationships.

Earlier I mentioned that you will glow effortlessly when you practice Give, Give, Get with those who are natural, kindred spirits. When I first began dating after my divorce, I got the best relationship advice from my therapist: "Angela, I coach my clients to use the love language tool when they are in a marriage that is stuck. However, my advice to you as you date is to find someone who speaks your love language. During times of stress, we revert to what comes naturally. If you and your partner have a shared love language, it gives you a natural advantage."

We can apply this "shared language" advice to all of our relationships. When what matters to us (a value, goal, ethos, or passion) is shared by others, relationships at home and at work will inevitably flow, and both people can give from a place of authenticity and alignment. This next ritual will help you give and get what matters.

⋆ RITUAL: Give and Get What Matters

To better understand what is essential to loved ones

Time: 10 minutes
Ingredients: Pen and paper or a digital device

Optional Upgrades: Candles, crystals, fresh rose
Notes: You can reflect on these thought starters, or
you can write your responses down in a journal.

1. **Ask**. During a chat with a loved one, friend, or
   coworker, you can ask the following questions to
   understand what's important to them:
   a. What does success look like to you?
   b. What do you value most in your life?
   c. What makes you feel safe and loved?
   d. What are your stressors?
   e. What's your love language?

2. **Awaken.** Become aware of what is essential to the
   other party, and if it feels right, honor it when it
   counts. For example, my daughter loves structure
   and wants to know her schedule, allowance,
   rewards, and responsibilities on paper. Even though
   I have a less structured approach to life, I try to give
   her this organization because it is what makes her
   feel safe and respected.

3. **Align.** You can also do this ritual with yourself to
   stay in your radiance and attract people who reflect
   your highest good, too. The answers can illuminate
   when it's time to let go of a relationship to keep the
   space open for the right one(s).

Give Grace

Forgiveness is a funny thing. It warms
the heart and cools the sting.
—William Arthur Ward, writer

Giving grace in relationships is about letting the small things go for the sake of the bigger vision or intention. We tend to think that forgiveness benefits the other person, but in reality, giving grace lightens our load, uplifts our spirits, and, frankly, I'm convinced it even diminishes stress wrinkles!

As a pianist, I was part of a chamber music group called Trio Movado. We had hours of rehearsals together in a practice room, and while there were many fun times, sometimes passionate pleas for a musical idea would escalate into an argument. Someone would stop in the middle of playing and begin to describe what she had envisioned: "Let's crescendo [get louder] before the end of the phrase." Then someone else would pipe in: "No, I disagree. It's much more atmospheric if we diminuendo [get softer]." Often, egos would inflate, and each musician would compete to prove who was right or wrong versus what best served the music.

One day, Julie, the cellist, said something so wise that it's stuck with me to today: "The words are getting in the way," she said. "Let's stop talking, start playing, and begin listening with more awareness. We will feel the intention, and things will fall into place naturally." Inevitably, the chatter and noise did die down, and the original musical intentions became apparent.

We don't always communicate our intentions in the best way, because sometimes our egos, and therefore, words, get in the way. We are often products of our past joys and hurt: when we feel heated, we may say things that don't serve our highest intentions and can sabotage our relationships. Giving grace means taking time to empathize with the other person's perspective and letting go of the words, for the sake of the bigger picture and relationship.

If, for example, you are experiencing tension with a coworker, I suggest that you get to the heart of the matter by letting go of what's being said and focusing instead on how each other's strengths contribute to the bigger goal. Or maybe, a text exchange with a loved one becomes negative due to a misunderstanding. Instead of assuming the worst, pick up the phone and give the benefit of the doubt to better understand the other side. When you give grace to heal an unnecessary fracture, your "Get" can be deeper awareness, compassionate understanding, and a more harmonious outcome.

RITUAL: Give Grace

To hear intention

Time: 10 minutes

Ingredients: Pen and paper or a digital device, face cream of choice

Optional Upgrades: Candle, crystal, soothing meditation music

1. **Breathe.** Inhale and exhale slowly until you feel grounded.
2. **Massage.** Take a pearl-sized amount of your favorite face cream and begin massaging your heart, décolletage, and neck area while saying the affirmation, *"I open my heart and let the tension melt away"* or *"I focus on the bigger picture."*
3. **Ask.** Reflect on a relationship that feels challenging. Ask yourself the following questions:
   a. What do I value most about this relationship? What's important to me?
   b. What is my intention in this particular situation? Could I communicate better without judgment or pointing fingers?
   c. What is his/her intention? Do I need to ask

to clarify? How can I better empathize and understand?

Important note: This is not about accepting or excusing abusive behavior. Please seek professional help if these boundaries are crossed.

4. **Affirm.** When you feel that words and ego are getting in the way, create an affirmation to recite, such as, *"I listen to my heart and act with wisdom."*

The "Awaken Awareness" section in week 6's "Create Your Radiant Vibration" is a beautiful complement to giving grace.

Give "Little Sweets"

It's always the little things, those little gestures, that matter the most.
—Unknown

Valentine's Day was approaching this past year, and I was getting nervous. It was the first year with my partner, and I didn't know what to expect. I confided to my hairdresser, Donnie, "I have no idea if he's planning on doing anything, so I don't want to be embarrassed if I get him a gift and he doesn't get me one or vice versa!" My partner is not American, and we were discovering, enjoying, and getting used to our cultural differences. Valentine's Day is a big deal in the United States, so I wanted to manage my expectations and protect my heart just in case. Donnie, the best advice giver (as so many hairdressers are!), encouraged me to bring up my thoughts so that we could align on how we would (or would not) celebrate; this would help both me and my partner avoid disappointment.

At dinner, I casually asked my partner if we should make dinner reservations somewhere since restaurants were getting booked up. He looked surprised and responded, "I'm not crazy about celebrating love on one day. We should treat every day like Valentine's Day and not just February 14. Why don't we focus on 'little sweets' every day? We make morning coffee for each other, give massages, and write gratitude notes every single day. In my opinion, these little moments are much more important than the big ones."

My partner then explained that he'd once been in a marriage full of surprise birthday parties and expensive gifts for anniversaries and birthdays, but the little daily things were never appreciated or celebrated. So even though he surprised me with red roses on February 14 after all, his "little sweets" philosophy was the more significant and impactful gift that keeps on giving.

Here are some "little sweets" that you can give to friends and family:

- Send a text sharing what you love about them.
- Leave a note with a compliment before leaving for the day.
- Venmo ten to twenty dollars with a "Lunch is on me!" inspirational message.
- Have a surprise picnic.
- Do an unexpected chore.
- Bring a treat to a meeting.
- Gift a friend your favorite new discovery, such as a hand cream or bath salts.
- Be the planner of your group and get everyone together for a day at the beach or park.
- Surprise a loved one with hard-to-get chocolate, candy, or specialty food.
- Set up a weekend "walk and talk" for some bonding time.

The richness of relationships lies in small gestures for friends, family, and loved ones—giving (and getting!) a hit of happiness—which is the best radiance elixir for all. Cheers to that!

RITUAL: Give "Little Sweets"

To give and get a hit of happy!

Time: 10+ minutes
Ingredients: Pen and paper or a digital device

1. List. Who would you like to appreciate? Write down their names (and don't forget yourself!).

2. Reflect. What are small ways that you could give "little sweets"? It doesn't have to be expensive to show appreciation! The best gifts are free, like sending text messages with a note of gratitude to friends or coworkers.

3. Give. Every time you give a "little sweet," say an affirmation to yourself like, *"I love giving from a cup that overflows!"*

Give, Give, *Get*

Love cures people—both the ones who give it and the ones who receive it.

—Dr. Karl A. Menninger

The "Get" in Give, Give, Get is about allowing and receiving. I've found that when you give from a full cup with good intentions, the universe then provides you with opportunities to receive great things in your life as a kind of goodwill payback or a balancing of scales.

Have you heard the saying that people come into your life for a reason, a season, or a lifetime? I always like to find the reason, and for me, this is the "Get" in Give, Give, Get. Receiving is as essential as giving, but this part of the cycle is where the energy gets stuck for most people. By not receiving from others, we don't allow them to contribute to the circle of giving, which is what helps make us humans thrive. Reciprocation is essential to this Give, Give, Get equation because it's what brings balance and true sustenance to a relationship. Without receiving, we don't experience the restorative energy of another person's love, empathy, and generosity, which are expressed through giving. When we receive, we allow others to complete their cycle of Give, Give, Get. It's as important for you as it is for them.

So how do we open ourselves to receive? We slow down, relax, and allow the other person to "drive the car," so to speak. I learned how to receive when I began dating after twenty years of marriage. At the time, my only real awareness of what it was like to date in New York City was informed by old reruns of *Sex and the City* and *Friends*. And more recently, I kept hearing from friends that New York City was a horrific dating jungle due to hectic work schedules and expensive outings. However, I decided that I would *get* a lot out of each date by approaching it as a fun, learning adventure. I would not control outcomes or conversations. I would not be the boss of the date. I would not judge the experience. I would let it all go. And even if there wasn't a second or third date, I knew I would, at the very least, learn something new and interesting. For instance, there were the following dates:

The entrepreneur who taught me how to cook a steak
The Frenchman who introduced me to fantastic Soho
   restaurants
The gynecologist who showed me how to appreciate
   bourbon
The Brooklyn surfer who helped me navigate Spotify
   playlists

Sometimes, *asking* for the "Get" is part of the process, too. We have all heard the saying, "Ask, and you shall receive." This reminds me of how, the other day, my friend Kat and I were chatting on the phone. We began to talk about cooking, and I discovered that she was a passionate amateur chef and baker. We drooled over our recent creations, from Nutella banana bread, pesto salad dressing, and Brazilian salmon stew, to a sticky toffee pudding recipe I'd just discovered at the Bluebird London restaurant in New York City. I told her that I loved it so much that we ordered a second plate, and I even mustered up the courage to ask the chef for the recipe.

To my delight, he hand-wrote the recipe for me. "Hey, if you don't ask, you'll never receive!" I said to her, and she piped in, "The worst they can say is no, and now I need to ask you for that recipe!" I promptly texted it to her, and she sent me her cashew-cilantro dip recipe in return—which she got from her friend Julie, and I'm now sharing it with you!

Kat's Cashew-Cilantro Dip

¼ cup olive oil

¼ cup soy sauce (I use gluten-free)

1 cup roasted, unsalted cashews

3 cloves garlic

1½ tablespoons sugar (I use coconut sugar)

2 tablespoons rice vinegar

1 tablespoon lemon juice

1 squeeze sriracha hot chili sauce

1 bunch cilantro, washed (stems okay)

Directions: Combine all ingredients in a blender until smooth and thick. Refrigerate before serving.

I hope you'll enjoy this delicious little "Get"! The following ritual will shift your mindset to open you up to receive even more "Gets" in the future.

RITUAL: Give, Give, Get

To receive with grace

Time: 10 minutes

Notes: This is a ritual you can practice wherever you go to receive.

1. **Breathe.** Start by breathing in and out in a relaxing rhythm. Think of a color that you find soothing. Imagine this color flowing through you and surrounding you.
2. **Soften.** When you are with others, refrain from overgiving, taking charge, or pushing an agenda. Notice your breath, allow the conversation to flow, and listen with intent.
3. **Absorb.** Observe whatever comes up in the conversation or interaction. Acknowledge what you receive when you learn something new, feel inspired, or are entertained.
4. **Receive.** What we are grateful for grows, so make sure to appreciate the takeaways and gifts!

Your Give, Give, Get Plan

1. **Schedule.** Plan some time with friends and family to start practicing the rituals in this chapter. With

every interaction, enjoy deepening your Give, Give, Get practice.

- LISTEN WITH YOUR EYES (to deepen connection with others)
- GIVE AND GET WHAT MATTERS (to understand what's important to others)
- GIVE GRACE (to focus on the bigger picture)
- GIVE "LITTLE SWEETS" (to increase "feel good" vibes)
- GIVE, GIVE, GET (to receive gifts from relationships)

2. Plan. Write in your planner or put in a GCal reminder when you will do these rituals. Remember that scheduling in rituals prioritizes *you*!

3. Cleanse. Don't forget to cleanse and hydrate your skin at night while saying your affirmations!

4. Affirm. Create three to five self-worth affirmations. Write them on sticky notes, in your journal, or add to your affirmations deck. For example:
"I give from a full cup. My cup overflows with love and generosity."

5. Love. Schedule a self-love activity that elevates your ability to give, give, *get*.

GLOW WITH GRATITUDE

We began our twelve-week self-love journey with skincare, which is where I first discovered the importance of radiant self-love. To treat your skin like the most expensive silk on earth, as my mom would say, is an honor that we've additionally applied to the soul throughout this book. Beauty creams and serums nourish our outer radiance, and now we've come full circle to the notion of gratitude, a healing balm that restores and renews our inner shine. What we appreciate *appreciates,* and when we bask in abundance, we radiate what I call the "gratitude glow."

A gratitude glow can take years off your face. When we live in the aura of appreciation, peace and beauty diminish stress lines and magnify youthful vibrancy. An attitude of gratitude can lift any burden off your shoulders so that you feel free, breathe easy, and walk with poise. So when you hurt, turn to gratitude. When you are angry, come back to gratitude. Soak and bask in the nourishment of appreciating the most basic things in life, like being able to see, walk, and breathe. Sometimes it is the last thing you'll want to do, but even if you have to say something as basic as, "I'm grateful that I have a roof over my head," gratitude will bring you home to love, which is where all sustainable decisions and actions are made.

As an example, many people have asked me how my ex-husband and I managed to divorce so amicably. The answer is that I am thankful. I am thankful for the good (and not-so-good) experiences we shared, because they prepared me for who I am today. Yes, of course, I went through a period of sadness and heartache. And while triggers from the past still exist, I have chosen to focus on the lessons and takeaways. What didn't resonate with me in my marriage illuminated what I desired, and this clarity is my golden guiding light. When past wounds resurface from time to time, I consider the Korean skin philosophy that deals with the root cause: I view these stressors as an opportunity to grow with awareness and heal from within. Hiding or ignoring the problems only robs me of self-growth, which is key to emotional freedom.

While dating in New York City, I heard countless stories of acrimonious interactions with ex-spouses. Not everyone is able to maintain a friendship with their ex, and I'm fortunate that my ex is reasonable and kind. So many ex-couples do not communicate directly, rack up costly attorney bills, use the police to hold the other person accountable for his or her behavior, and put their kids in the middle of already-uncomfortable conversations as confidantes and messengers. In most cases, vitriol and blame become the crutches they use to hobble out of a toxic environment.

In chapter 9, I shared one of my favorite quotes with you by Mizuta Masahide, a seventeenth-century Japanese poet and samurai, that goes, "Barn's burnt down—now I can see the moon." Isn't that lovely? When the chips are down and we choose to live by this adage, we have the opportunity to gain clarity. This is why I did not view my divorce as an end or failure. I looked up and saw the marvelous moon instead. The end of my relationship was a new beginning; I appreciated the chance to clean up my side of the street. I was given a second chance to discover who I am and honor authenticity.

In any life situation, we have choices: we can choose to feel robbed, angry, or depleted during conflicts, or we can allow gratitude to continually restore and renew our spirits. Our souls sing freely when we let go of the past, the weight of the present, and the worries of the future. To live in gratitude is to fully enjoy, relish, and savor the abundance in and around us. It's a way of being, and your gratitude glow will magnetize a lifetime of momentous, radiant miracles ahead.

Future-Self Gratitude

Self-love is an action for which your
future self will thank you.
—**Angela Jia Kim**

The original mission behind Savor Beauty was to help our clients renew and restore skin radiance. I didn't expect that our ethos would eventually deepen and expand into a profound philosophy of soul radiance. Through self-love, we have discovered an elusive beauty secret. When we layer love and nourishment onto our inner and outer selves with soothing balms and rituals, we gain the clarity and courage to choose authenticity over approval. We can then make choices from a place of wholeness and integrity.

Self-love is an action for which our future selves will thank us. Knowing this, we need to talk about taking action that comes from our highest intentions—i.e., those that are underscored by integrity. When most people think about integrity, they view it from a religious, moralistic, or self-righteous perspective: when you don't behave with integrity, it's judged as sinning or doing something wrong. Author Martha Beck, however, defines integrity more holistically. She says it's acting in a way that allows you to be one, whole, and undivided. To illustrate this point, she says we need emotional and behavioral integrity to function in the same way that an airplane needs structural integrity to fly. Beck says that if even one piece of us is out of alignment, there's internal division; the plane, or our lives, can crash.

When we don't act with integrity, we disconnect from our spirit and can sabotage our amazing life force. Stagnation, depression, illness, and fragmentation can arise from this and ultimately destroy our lives. But when we uphold our integrity, we radiate our authentic truth and beauty so that our lives can flourish. We make hundreds of decisions every day, and when we make them with our whole selves, we act according to our highest intentions and for the good of all. Not only do we make better choices this way, but we also make the *right* choices to feed the bliss and balance we desire. To stay in this optimal state, we need to continually nurture our radiance and take care of the bits and pieces that make us whole.

How do we know if we are honoring our integrity? Here are five rules I try to live by:

1. I make agreements and honor them with others and myself.
2. I am honest in all of my communications and don't feel the need to lie.

3. I surround myself with people of integrity; like attracts (and influences) like!

4. I treat myself, others, and my surroundings with respect.

5. I invest my time and money responsibly.

Commit today to align and act from a place of integrity and gratitude. Your future self will stand in deep and humble gratitude for the miracles that are coming your way. Keep these words in mind as you embark on your journey of authenticity and integrity: *I am whole. I nourish my radiance with self-love every day. And I am grateful for the miracles coming my way.*

RITUAL: Savor Beauty

To stay in integrity with your highest self

Time: 10 minutes

Notes: I like to do this ritual before doing anything that may sabotage my integrity, whether it's eating non-nourishing foods or doing business with someone that feels out of alignment. It helps me to pause and make a better choice in the moment.

1. **Awaken.** As you make choices throughout the day, become more aware: Are you acting from a place of wholeness and integrity?

2. **Pause.** Notice your breath and see if you can slow down the inhalations and exhalations.

3. **Reflect.** Ask yourself, "What is the vibration of this action? Will my future self thank me?"

4. **Reset.** If you are not acting in integrity, what can you do instead to reflect your whole self? Replacing a lower-vibration action with a higher-vibration action on the spot is the best way to go from a divided self to a whole one. Consider going on a Radiance Retreat to raise your vibration and get back in alignment. Or read an affirmation from your affirmations deck.

5. **Appreciate.** Say an affirmation, such as, *"My future self thanks me for acting in integrity"* or *"I make decisions that are in alignment with my highest self for my highest good."*

Manifest Gratitude

Gratitude . . . turns what we have into enough, and more. It turns denial into acceptance, chaos to order, confusion to

clarity. . . . It . . . makes sense of our past, brings peace for today, and creates a vision for tomorrow.
—Melody Beattie, author

I have a secret manifesting trick that helps magnetize a desire: be grateful for it *before* it comes to fruition.

For four years, my Upper West Side apartment was my cozy retreat from the world, and I enjoyed every inch of it when my daughter and I were holed up during the COVID-19 lockdown. I called it our luxury treehouse next to Central Park, with its seventeen-foot ceilings, massive windows that flooded the living room with warmth and light, and hidden nooks and crannies that made it a "hide and seek" treasure for my daughter. Even so, there came a time when my growing tween needed more space, and I needed more privacy, so I put my place on the market.

Initially, my real estate agent said she'd never seen such a frenzy of inquiries, and she showed it to a flurry of enthusiastic buyers. Yet after four months, we did not receive one offer. This told me that something was energetically off. Whether I was not ready to part with the space or the timing wasn't right, I knew that a vibrational shift needed to occur. So I took the apartment off the market for a month and relisted it with another agent. This second time around, I meditated on feeling grateful for the abundance and ease of a fast sale. Every time I imagined the broker coming to me with an all-cash offer, I would say to myself, "I'm so grateful for abundance and ease." Wouldn't you know that a week after putting it on the market again, a Montana woman, who had only seen it over FaceTime, offered all-cash for my asking price?

It's important to trust in divine timing, and it's not always easy to feel grateful for something you are waiting for. Let's try a ritual that will help you manifest with appreciation.

RITUAL: Gratitude Manifestation

To call in manifestations with gratitude

Time: 10 minutes

Ingredients: Quiet space

Optional Upgrades: Crystals, essential oil, or an aromatic object (can be a candle, chocolate, coffee, basil leaf, etc.)

Notes: Remember to focus on how you want to feel versus the *specific* manifestation. For example, instead of focusing on the sale of the apartment, I felt abundance due to an easy sale.

1. Breathe. Inhale the scent you've chosen on a count of three, filling your belly, chest, and décolletage area. Exhale on a count of six, allowing your

décolletage, chest, and belly to decompress. Repeat
until you feel a sense of peace and calm.

2. Clarify. Choose the desired manifestation and,
more importantly, how you want to feel.

3. Affirm. Create an affirmation, such as, *"I am
grateful for the* [add feeling] *I feel from the* [add
manifestation]*"* or *"I am grateful for the abundance I
feel from the easy sale of the apartment."*

4. Appreciate. Imagine the feeling of gratitude
filling you up from your toes to your head.
Allow appreciation to swirl in and around you
until you feel grateful for the feeling you clarified
in step 2.

Share Gratitude

*At times, our own light goes out and is rekindled by a spark
from another person. Each of us has cause to think with deep
gratitude of those who have lighted the flame within us.*

—Albert Schweitzer, doctor and Nobel Peace Prize winner

Sharing our appreciation freely with loved ones illuminates and ignites a contagious gratitude glow. Appreciation was rarely expressed to me, having grown up in
a Korean household and during my time as a concert
pianist. Constant criticism was a method of motivation

to strive for excellence and perfection. When I became a professional pianist, harsh criticism became my guiding force. I would focus on the one missed note and disregard every other magical moment of a performance. Even when others expressed appreciation, I could not receive it; I was so intent on seeing the negative.

It's no surprise that I often fall back on this mindset if I'm not careful about it. I tend to look for "what's wrong" so that I can fix the issue and make it better. This theme runs through all aspects of my life, including my relationships. I recently decided, then, that it was time to break the pattern—and I began with my love life. Instead of focusing on a random negative comment that I might hear from my partner and blowing it out of proportion, I decided that I would focus on all the warm and uplifting things he says instead. To do this, I started a "Relationship Gratitude" note on my iPhone. Anytime my partner said or did something uplifting, I stored it in my phone. Over the course of a month, I amassed a list of over one hundred sweet things he said and did. As I read the list and felt gratitude, something magical happened; the negative lost its power on me, and the vibration of our relationship elevated.

When I showed my partner the gratitude list that I created, he loved it and said, "I want to do this practice with you." We decided to create a joint "Relationship Gratitude" note on our iPhones, and we make it a regular practice to write down what we appreciate about each other and about our lives. It feels so good to give, give, get appreciation, and now we also have a running document of shared experiences and memories.

If you like this idea, feel free to give it a try and even add your own twist. Perhaps start a family gratitude book or journal that you share among family members. You can end celebrations, vacations, gatherings, or special times by asking them to write anything they loved about the time you spent together. Then sit back to experience a mega gratitude glow.

RITUAL: Share Gratitude

To see your gratitude garden grow abundantly

Time: 3–5 minutes
Ingredients: Pen and journal or sticky notes, or the Notes app on your phone
Notes: You can use a journal for this ritual or the Notes app on your smartphone to share with your kids, partner, friends, or coworkers.

1. **Jot.** Whenever you feel thankful for something that someone did, jot it down, no matter how big or small.

2. Share. Make sure that the other persons see your appreciation, and come up with a system so that you can regularly give, give, get appreciation.

3. Scan. From time to time, reread this list to sit in the aura of appreciation.

4. Affirm. Create an affirmation, such as, *"I bask in the aura of appreciation"* or *"I love sharing gratitude with loved ones."*

Gratitude Gatherings

Two kinds of gratitude: The sudden kind we feel for what we take; the larger kind we feel for what we give.

—Edwin Arlington Robinson, poet

Over the years, I've come to notice that you can shift the energy of a group so that everyone experiences a collective gratitude glow—and all through the power of giving thanks. When the spa was planning its annual holiday party a few years ago, my West Village spa manager said that she had a hard time finding a time that worked for the team. The evening-shift team members didn't want to have a morning holiday brunch because they would have to come into the city and stick around for their shift. The morning-shift team members didn't want an evening party for the same reason. I felt disheartened at the lack of the holiday spirit and cheer.

Rather than call off the gathering, I decided to invite the entire team to a Thanksgiving gratitude brunch. We'd meet in the morning, and instead of gifts, each person would pick a random name out of a hat and give gratitude to that person. Much to my delight, there were no complaints, and everyone RSVP'd.

After placing our orders at the restaurant, my team and I went around the table to share our gratitude for each person. One person said, "One day, I came to work after receiving a health scare from my doctor. Even though I kept it to myself, you gave me an extra big hug that morning, and I felt so much love and support that it helped me get through the day." Another gushed, "What I appreciate about you is that you never just leave after your work is done. You always ask us if you can help with anything, and this creates such an amazing work culture for everyone. Thank you." The group's energy rose with stories that made us laugh and cry. As appreciation flowed, so did the good cheer—and each person beamed from the inside out.

Try this ritual with friends or family at your next gathering and watch their energy ignite a collective gratitude glow.

RITUAL: Gratitude Gathering

To illuminate group glow

Time: 5+ minutes

Ingredients: Two or more people

Notes: This is an excellent team or group activity or a fun dinner game. Tell everyone to come prepared to share something they appreciate about a designated person. I usually send a message like, "We're playing a fun little appreciation game at dinner! Please come prepared to share something you appreciate, admire, or are grateful for about person X."

1. **Share.** Set the stage by saying that everyone will share appreciation about a designated person in the room. You can break the ice by going first.
2. **Exchange.** Allow everyone in the room to share gratitude statements or stories.
3. **Appreciate.** In the end, you can close the ritual with a personal "thank you" to everyone.
4. **Savor.** Enjoy the gratitude glow that will uplift everyone present!

The Gratitude Glow

The more grateful I am, the more beauty I see.
—**Mary Davis, author**

During our self-love journey in this book, you learned that to cleanse your face every night is a profound act of supreme self-love. You learned to breathe in the aroma, massage away the day's tension, soften the skin, and sweep away dirt and toxins. Hopefully, you have experienced how ending every night with a face-cleansing ritual renews and replenishes both skin and soul.

That being said, there's one last Radiance Ritual that I want you to end your day with: yes, you guessed it—the Gratitude Glow.

One morning, I asked my daughter, Sienna, what she's learned most from me, and she said, "how to be grateful." I instantly melted, as I realized that all my lessons about the importance of being thankful hadn't fallen on deaf ears. They'd been planted in her little heart.

Perhaps this is because my daughter and I have always played a gratitude game when I tuck her into bed at night. We say three things that we're grateful for: one about each other, one about ourselves, and one about anything else. For a while, she'd say, "I'm thankful for Zoe" (our dog), and end there. So I came up with a formula to help her *feel* deeper appreciation: what I love + why I love it = how it makes me feel. Her gratitude statements became more heartfelt: "I love mama because she is caring. She made s'mores with me tonight, and I felt special."

Finally, we like to end our bedtime ritual with a statement of self-gratitude and self-love by saying one thing that we love about ourselves. One night, she said, "I love myself because today when the teacher said I didn't do the homework, I showed her evidence that I did it, and she apologized to me. I felt proud to stand up for myself even though I was nervous."

Yes, there are days when I feel like I can do better as a mom. But then there are moments like these when we both go to bed glowing with gratitude, and I can't think of a better self-love ritual to pass on to my little one.

My hope is that you, too, will embrace the Gratitude Glow as often as you can, as you manifest a radically radiant life filled with abundance, beauty, and joy.

RITUAL: Gratitude Glow

To go to bed glowing with gratitude

Time: 5 minutes

Notes: Do this ritual before going to bed by yourself or with a loved one!

1. **What.** State what you love, enjoy, admire, or something for which you feel gratitude.
2. **Why.** Be as descriptive as possible. Why do you love it or why do you feel grateful? Relish, enjoy, savor!
3. **Feel.** How does it make you feel? Wear this radiant feeling to end the day with the Gratitude Glow.

Your Gratitude Plan

1. **Schedule.** Carve out time for your self-love rituals, and make yourself a priority so you can give from a cup that overflows with peace and beauty.
   - SAVOR BEAUTY (to stay in integrity with your highest self)
   - GRATITUDE MANIFESTATION (to call in manifestations with gratitude)
   - SHARE GRATITUDE (to see your gratitude garden grow)
   - GRATITUDE GATHERING (to illuminate group glow)
   - GRATITUDE GLOW (to go to bed glowing with gratitude)
2. **Plan.** Write in your planner or put in a GCal reminder when you will do these rituals. Remember that scheduling in rituals prioritizes *you*!
3. **Cleanse.** Don't forget to cleanse and hydrate your skin at night while saying your affirmations!
4. **Affirm.** Create three to five gratitude affirmations.

Write them on sticky notes, in your journal, or add to your affirmations deck. For example:

"What I'm grateful for grows!"

5. Love. Schedule a self-love activity that elevates your gratitude and appreciation.

ACKNOWLEDGMENTS

I am deeply grateful to those who brought light to the messages in this book. Thank you for supporting me through this humbling journey, which has been a lifetime in the making.

Thank you to my editors at St. Martin's Press, Daniela Rapp and Cassidy Graham. Daniela, you saw the need and space for self-love and ignited the fire. Cassidy, you wrapped it in a beautiful bow to give the gift of radiance to our readers.

To my agent, Laura Nolan, who saw the spark from the start: thank you for encouraging me to dig deeper and for valuing the life experience I took for granted. And thank you to Danielle Zacharia for connecting the stars in the sky.

Thank you to Kristina Grish for bringing this book to life with me. I'm in awe of your ease and fluidity with words. You are one of the most gifted souls with whom I've been so fortunate to have worked. Thank you to Brynn Strugger for helping me refine Savor Beauty's message of self-love. Your style, substance, and sparkle are in every chapter.

To the beautiful team at Savor Beauty: your dedication to bringing beauty to all parts of the world inspired this book. A special thank-you to Escarla Abreu for creative art direction and to Samantha Hassel for refining the skin content.

Mom, thank you for mesmerizing me with your shiny skin and for being a beacon of generosity. Thank you to Dad for always looking out for us from above. Whenever you whispered into my ear, "I believe in you," I was invincible, and these words still bring me strength today. Thank you to my sisters, Emily and Joyce, for surviving, thriving, and living your dreams. I know Dad is beaming with pride. Thank you to Papant for being a quiet and formidable source of wisdom for us all. And thank you, Marc, for being my forever friend and co-parent and for the two decades of unforgettable delicious dinners.

To the women whose friendships I cherish: many of your stories and wisdom are in this book as a source of inspiration for others. Thank you to Sara Blette, Julie Kim, Victoria Lynden, Traci Bild, Kat Gordon, Kayle Koepke, Julie Albers, Rebecca Casciano, and to the Savor community. I am so grateful to you all for doing the deep work of going within and shining your radiance into my life.

My sweet love, Ali: thank you for seeing the halo from the first day. When I said to you, "no expectations or limitations," I had no idea of the abundance of limitless, juicy life experiences we would experience together. Here's to soulmate magic, dancing our hearts out, and going deep and wide with all the love found in pink sunrises, red sunsets, turquoise oceans, bright stars, and double rainbows.

To the light of my life, Sisi: from the day that you kissed a chocolate-chip cookie and declared it your best friend, I knew that you would remind me to cherish everything sweet in life. You gave me so much love and creativity from the time you were a one-month-old in my arms, helping me sell creams in the cold, and I will give love and strength back to you all the days of my life.

And thank you, dear reader, for nourishing your radiance. Your lit-from-within love is seen, felt, and appreciated.

Thank you, thank you, thank you.

ABOUT THE AUTHOR

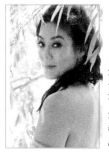

Credit: Lisa-Marie Mazzucco

ANGELA JIA KIM is the founder of Savor Beauty, a natural skincare and facial spa brand inspired by Korean beauty and self-love rituals, and a former international, classical concert pianist. Called "the unexpected beauty virtuoso" by MindBodyGreen, she created the award-winning skincare in her kitchen, became an accidental entrepreneur, and built a multimillion-dollar enterprise around the philosophy of manifesting beauty, brilliance, and balance. She has led hundreds of women empowerment workshops and her *Savor Beauty Planner* has sold over 100,000 copies. Her skincare and spas in New York City have been chosen as "Best of New York" and featured in top publications such as *Vogue*, *goop*, *Elle*, *Allure*, and *InStyle*.

Angela lives in New York City.